Preface

Health, both physical and mental, has always been at the core of my personal and professional journey. I pursued a degree in Psychological Sciences, followed by a diploma in Naturopathy and certification as a Personal Trainer. These three areas form the foundation of my holistic approach to health, which treats the body and mind as interconnected elements, each essential to achieving a deep and lasting balance.

What started as a passion for physical and mental well-being naturally evolved into a focus on nutrition. Over time, I came to understand that what we eat not only affects our physical shape but also profoundly influences our mental state, energy levels, and how we face daily challenges.

It's important to clarify from the outset that this book is not intended as a medical guide, nor is it meant to replace professional advice. Any decisions regarding your health should always be made in consultation with your trusted physician. Through these pages, I aim to share the knowledge and practical experience I've accumulated over years of studying naturopathy, psychology, and fitness, offering a foundation for how nutrition, stress management, and lifestyle choices can enhance overall well-being.

This book is designed for a wide audience: health professionals, holistic doctors, naturopaths, wellness practitioners, and anyone seeking to better understand their body. My approach is built on an integrated vision of health, where nutrition, stress management, physical activity, and mental care work together to promote long-term wellness.

Throughout my studies, I've had the opportunity to dive deep into various disciplines—from the workings of the nervous system and human emotions to the physiology of the body and natural therapies. I've spent countless hours studying to develop a comprehensive understanding of health, and this book is my way of sharing that knowledge with those who, like me, believe in the importance of caring for themselves in a mindful and holistic way.

The heart of this book is about nutrition and its impact on metabolism, hormonal balance, and mental health. But it doesn't stop there: I also explore how stress, sleep, physical activity, and the environment play crucial roles in shaping our overall well-being. There are no universal answers, as each individual is different, and what works for one person may not work for another. My goal is to provide you with the tools to better understand your own body and make informed, personalized choices.

Health is a journey, not a destination. I hope that these pages provide you with new insights to navigate that journey with greater awareness and peace of mind. Even the smallest positive changes can have a significant impact on your overall well-being.

I extend my deepest thanks to everyone who has supported me along the way, especially my family and colleagues, who have always believed in the value of this work. I hope this book serves as a practical guide to improving your health and accompanies you on the path to a more balanced and mindful life.

INTRODUCTION

Introduction to Metabolic Health

Metabolic health plays a vital role in our overall well-being and encompasses the complex biochemical processes that allow our bodies to convert food into energy. This transformation is not merely a mechanical function; it significantly influences how we feel, think, and live our daily lives. A well-functioning metabolism ensures that our bodies can efficiently manage energy production, regulate blood sugar levels, and store or utilize fat appropriately. Understanding metabolic health requires a comprehensive view of how various factors, such as diet, exercise, and sleep, interact within our bodies. These elements are interconnected, and a disturbance in one can ripple through to affect the others. For instance, inadequate sleep can lead to insulin resistance, a precursor to type 2 diabetes, while a poor diet can fuel inflammation and disrupt hormonal balance. This book aims to illuminate these relationships, offering insights that empower you to take control of your metabolic health. Metabolic health is increasingly recognized as a key determinant of longevity and quality of life. Research suggests that maintaining metabolic balance can reduce the risk of various chronic diseases, including heart disease, diabetes, and obesity. By prioritizing metabolic health, you are not only investing in a longer life but also in a life filled with energy and vitality.

Importance of Being Aware of Your Health Status

In our fast-paced society, health often takes a backseat until problems arise. Many individuals ignore early warning signs of metabolic dysfunction—such as fatigue, mood swings, and weight gain—assuming these symptoms are merely part of aging or stress. However, adopting a proactive approach to health can significantly alter the trajectory of your life. Being aware of your metabolic health involves regularly monitoring key biomarkers, such as blood glucose, cholesterol levels, and body composition. Understanding these markers can help you identify potential health risks before they escalate into serious issues. This awareness empowers you to make informed choices regarding your nutrition, exercise, and lifestyle habits. Incorporating simple, routine health checks can foster a sense of control over your well-being. For example, tracking your dietary intake, exercise routines, and sleep patterns can help you identify areas for improvement. Knowledge is power, and being informed about your metabolic status enables you to make changes that positively impact your health. This awareness cultivates a deeper connection to your body. When you understand how your body responds to certain foods, activities, and stressors, you can create a personalized approach to wellness that aligns with your individual needs. The journey towards improved health begins with understanding your unique metabolic profile.

Goals of the Book

This book is structured as a comprehensive guide to improving your metabolic health, offering insights, practical tools, and motivation for readers at all stages of their health journeys. The primary goals are:

1.   **Educate:** To provide clear, accessible information about metabolic health and its relevance to everyday life. Complex scientific concepts will be broken down into understandable terms, ensuring that readers from various backgrounds can grasp the material.

2.   **Empower:** To equip readers with practical strategies for monitoring and enhancing their metabolic health. From dietary changes to exercise recommendations, the book will provide actionable steps to help readers take control of their well-being.

3.   **Inspire:** To share success stories and testimonials that demonstrate the positive impact of improving metabolic health. These narratives will serve as motivation and encouragement, showing readers that change is not only possible but achievable.

4.   **Support:** To offer a structured plan that includes resources, recipes, and guidelines for implementing lifestyle changes effectively. The book will serve as a roadmap, guiding readers through the complexities of health improvement while fostering a sense of community.

5.   **Engage:** To involve readers in their health journey by encouraging self-reflection and active participation. Questions, exercises, and interactive components will prompt readers to engage with the material on a deeper level. By the end of this book, you will have a comprehensive understanding of metabolic health and the tools needed to make informed decisions about your well-being. This journey is not just about avoiding illness; it is about thriving and living a fulfilling life. Your path to optimal health starts here, and together, we will explore the intricate connections that define your metabolic health.

1. UNDERSTANDING METABOLISM

1.1 The Science of Metabolism

Definition of Metabolism

Metabolism is the sum of all biochemical processes that occur within a living organism to maintain life. It involves the conversion of food into energy, allowing cells to perform vital functions essential for survival. Metabolism is generally categorized into two main components: catabolism and anabolism.

•**Catabolism** refers to the breakdown of complex molecules into simpler ones, releasing energy in the process. For instance, carbohydrates consumed in our diet are broken down into glucose, which serves as a primary energy source for cells. This breakdown not only provides immediate energy but also supplies the building blocks necessary for various cellular functions.

•**Anabolism**, in contrast, involves the synthesis of larger molecules from smaller ones, a process that requires energy. This phase of metabolism is critical for growth, repair, and maintenance of tissues. For example, amino acids are assembled into proteins, which are essential for muscle repair and various biochemical functions within the body.

Metabolism operates continuously, adapting to the body's needs based on factors like physical activity, dietary intake, and hormonal balance. Understanding how metabolism works is crucial for recognizing its role in health, fitness, and overall well-being.

Cellular Functions and Energy Production

At the cellular level, metabolism is fundamental for a wide array of processes, including growth, reproduction, and response to environmental changes. Each cell requires a constant supply of energy to sustain its activities, which include nutrient transport, waste removal, and communication with other cells. The primary mechanism for energy production in cells is called **cellular respiration**. This multi-step process can be summarized in three main stages:

1.   **Glycolysis**: This initial stage occurs in the cytoplasm of the cell, where glucose is broken down into two molecules of pyruvate. This process generates a small

yield of ATP (adenosine triphosphate), which cells use for energy. Glycolysis does not require oxygen, making it an anaerobic process.

2.   **Krebs Cycle**: Also known as the citric acid cycle, this stage occurs in the mitochondria. The pyruvate from glycolysis is further oxidized to produce carbon dioxide, and in the process, additional ATP, as well as electron carriers like NADH and $FADH_2$, are generated. These carriers are crucial for the next phase of energy production.

3.   **Electron Transport Chain (ETC)**: In this final stage, the electrons from NADH and $FADH_2$ are transferred through a series of protein complexes located in the inner mitochondrial membrane. As electrons move along the chain, they release energy, which is used to pump protons into the mitochondrial intermembrane space. This creates a proton gradient that drives the synthesis of a large amount of ATP through a process called oxidative phosphorylation. Oxygen acts as the final electron acceptor, forming water as a byproduct. The efficiency of energy production is influenced by several factors, including the type of nutrients consumed, physical activity levels, and overall metabolic health. Regular exercise, for example, can enhance mitochondrial function, increasing the body's ability to produce energy efficiently.

Role of Enzymes in Metabolism

Enzymes are specialized proteins that catalyze biochemical reactions in the body, playing an essential role in metabolism. They facilitate various metabolic processes by lowering the activation energy required for reactions to occur. Without enzymes, many metabolic reactions would proceed too slowly to support life. The role of enzymes in metabolism can be outlined as follows:

●**Catalysis**: Enzymes speed up metabolic reactions by providing an alternative pathway that requires less energy. Each enzyme is specific to a particular reaction or group of reactions, allowing for precise control over metabolic pathways.

●**Regulation**: Enzyme activity can be influenced by various factors, including substrate availability, temperature, pH levels, and the presence of inhibitors or activators. This regulation allows the body to adapt to changing conditions and energy demands. For instance, during periods of fasting, certain enzymes are upregulated to promote the breakdown of stored fats for energy.

●**Coenzymes and Cofactors**: Many enzymes require additional non-protein molecules, known as coenzymes or cofactors, to function effectively. These can include vitamins and minerals that assist in enzymatic activity. For example, B vitamins serve as coenzymes in energy metabolism, highlighting the importance of a balanced diet in supporting metabolic health.

Enzymatic reactions are tightly regulated to ensure metabolic balance. Disruptions in enzyme function can lead to metabolic disorders and health issues. For example, genetic mutations affecting enzyme production can result in conditions such as phenylketonuria (PKU), where the body cannot metabolize the amino acid phenylalanine, leading to toxic buildup.

Furthermore, understanding the dynamics of enzymes provides insights into how lifestyle choices impact metabolism. For instance, dietary choices that promote enzyme efficiency, such as consuming whole foods rich in nutrients, can enhance metabolic processes and overall health. Metabolism is a complex network of biochemical reactions that sustain life. By understanding its fundamental principles, individuals can make informed decisions that optimize their metabolic health, leading to improved energy levels, better weight management, and a reduced risk of chronic diseases. Embracing a holistic approach to metabolic health involves recognizing the interconnectedness of diet, physical activity, and lifestyle factors that collectively influence our well-being.

1.2 Key Biomarkers of Health

Types of Biomarkers

Biomarkers are measurable indicators of biological processes, health conditions, or responses to interventions. In the context of metabolic health, certain biomarkers provide valuable insights into how well the body is functioning at a cellular level. Understanding these biomarkers is crucial for identifying potential health risks and making informed lifestyle choices.

The key types of biomarkers relevant to metabolic health include:

●**Metabolic Markers**: These include glucose, insulin, and lipid profiles. Elevated blood glucose levels can indicate insulin resistance, a precursor to type 2 diabetes. Monitoring cholesterol levels, including LDL (bad cholesterol) and HDL (good cholesterol), can provide insights into cardiovascular health. For example, a high LDL level is associated with an increased risk of atherosclerosis, while higher HDL levels are generally protective.

•**Inflammatory Markers**: Chronic inflammation is linked to various metabolic disorders. Biomarkers like C-reactive protein (CRP) and interleukin-6 (IL-6) can help assess inflammation levels in the body, signaling potential risks for conditions such as heart disease and obesity. Regular monitoring of these markers can guide dietary and lifestyle changes aimed at reducing inflammation.

•**Hormonal Markers**: Hormones play a significant role in regulating metabolism. For example, thyroid hormones (T3 and T4) influence metabolic rate, while cortisol levels can indicate stress response and its impact on metabolism. Monitoring these hormones can provide a clearer picture of metabolic health, especially in relation to weight management and energy levels.

•**Oxidative Stress Markers**: Oxidative stress results from an imbalance between free radicals and antioxidants in the body. Biomarkers such as malondialdehyde (MDA) and 8-hydroxydeoxyguanosine (8-OHdG) can indicate the extent of oxidative damage, which is linked to various chronic diseases, including cancer and neurodegenerative disorders.

Understanding these biomarkers allows individuals to assess their metabolic health and take proactive steps to improve it.

How to Measure Metabolic Health

Measuring metabolic health involves assessing the key biomarkers discussed above. Various methods can be employed to obtain accurate readings, enabling individuals to monitor their health status effectively.

1.   **Blood Tests**: Blood tests are the most common method for measuring metabolic biomarkers. These tests can provide comprehensive profiles, including glucose levels, lipid panels, and inflammatory markers. For instance, a fasting blood glucose test can reveal how well your body manages sugar, while a lipid panel will help you understand your cholesterol levels. Regular blood work can help track changes over time and identify potential issues early on. It is recommended to discuss these results with a healthcare provider to create a personalized health plan.

2.   **Home Monitoring Devices**: With advancements in technology, several devices are now available for home monitoring. Glucose meters allow individuals with diabetes to keep track of their blood sugar levels, while continuous glucose monitors (CGMs) provide real-time data throughout the day. Smart scales can measure body composition, giving insights into muscle mass and body fat percentage. These devices enable individuals to track their metabolic health conveniently and adjust their lifestyles as needed.

3.   **Wearable Technology**: Fitness trackers and smartwatches can monitor various physiological parameters, including heart rate, sleep patterns, and physical activity levels. For example, devices that monitor heart rate variability (HRV) can provide insights into how well your body is managing stress. By analyzing this data, individuals can gain insights into their metabolic health and identify areas for improvement. Many of these devices also offer integration with health apps, providing a comprehensive overview of health metrics.

4.   **Urine Tests**: Some metabolic markers can also be assessed through urine analysis. For instance, measuring ketones can provide insights into fat metabolism, particularly for those following ketogenic diets. Urinary analysis can also reveal hydration status, which is crucial for metabolic function. By evaluating these parameters, individuals can better understand their metabolic state and make informed dietary choices.

5.   **Genetic Testing**: Genetic tests can provide information about inherited traits that may influence metabolic health. For instance, certain genetic markers may predispose individuals to conditions like obesity or insulin resistance. Understanding one's genetic predisposition can guide personalized lifestyle changes and health strategies. Genetic testing can be particularly useful for tailoring diet and exercise plans to individual needs, optimizing metabolic health based on one's unique genetic profile.

Taking a proactive approach to measuring metabolic health empowers individuals to stay informed and take charge of their well-being.

Interpreting Results

Once metabolic health biomarkers are measured, interpreting the results accurately is crucial for understanding one's health status and potential risks. Here are some key considerations when analyzing biomarker data:

•**Reference Ranges**: Most laboratory tests provide reference ranges, indicating what is considered normal for healthy individuals. However, these ranges can vary based on factors such as age, sex, and health status. For example, normal fasting glucose levels are generally between 70-99 mg/dL, but what is considered optimal can differ based on individual health conditions. It is important to discuss results with a healthcare provider to understand how they apply to individual circumstances.

•**Trends Over Time**: One isolated test result may not provide a complete picture of metabolic health. Tracking biomarker levels over time can reveal trends that may indicate improving or worsening health conditions. For instance, a gradual increase in fasting blood glucose levels may suggest a developing insulin resistance. This longitudinal perspective is vital for making informed lifestyle changes and adjusting health strategies accordingly.

•**Holistic Context**: It is essential to consider the overall health context when interpreting results. A high cholesterol level may be concerning, but if an individual is physically active and has a healthy lifestyle, it may require a different approach than someone with a sedentary lifestyle. Factors such as diet, exercise, stress, and sleep all play a role in metabolic health. Evaluating these aspects can provide a more comprehensive understanding of health.

•**Collaborative Approach**: Engaging with healthcare professionals, such as doctors or nutritionists, can provide valuable insights into interpreting results. These experts can help individuals understand their biomarkers in relation to their overall health goals and recommend appropriate interventions or lifestyle modifications. They can also assist in developing personalized plans that incorporate dietary adjustments, exercise routines, and stress management techniques.

•**Setting Goals**: Understanding biomarker results can empower individuals to set realistic health goals. Whether it involves adjusting dietary habits, increasing physical activity, or managing stress, having clear objectives can enhance motivation and lead to positive health outcomes. For instance, if cholesterol levels are elevated, an individual might aim to incorporate more heart-healthy foods, such as omega-3 fatty acids, into their diet.

In conclusion, recognizing and understanding key biomarkers of health is essential for optimizing metabolic function and overall well-being. By measuring these biomarkers, interpreting the results, and taking informed actions, individuals can actively manage their health and reduce the risk of chronic diseases.

1.3 Common Roots of Diseases

Correlation Between Metabolism and Chronic Diseases

Metabolism is the foundation of our body's energy management and overall health. A dysfunctional metabolic process can lead to various chronic diseases. At its core, metabolism involves how our bodies convert food into energy, regulate hormone levels, and manage waste. When these processes are disrupted, it can result in conditions such as obesity, type 2 diabetes, cardiovascular diseases, and metabolic syndrome.

Research shows that poor metabolic health significantly increases the risk of developing chronic diseases. For example, insulin resistance, where cells become less responsive to insulin, can lead to elevated blood sugar levels, contributing to type 2 diabetes. Similarly, metabolic dysregulation can affect lipid metabolism, leading to high levels of LDL cholesterol and increasing cardiovascular risks. Understanding these correlations allows us to see the broader picture of health, emphasizing the importance of maintaining optimal metabolic function.

Examples of Related Conditions

1. **Obesity**: Obesity is often rooted in metabolic dysfunction, where an imbalance between calorie intake and expenditure leads to excessive fat accumulation. This condition is linked to numerous health problems, including type 2 diabetes, hypertension, and certain cancers.

2. **Type 2 Diabetes**: This condition stems from insulin resistance, which is a direct consequence of poor metabolic health. Elevated blood sugar levels can cause various complications, including nerve damage, kidney disease, and cardiovascular issues.

3. **Cardiovascular Diseases**: Conditions such as heart disease and stroke are closely tied to metabolic health. High levels of cholesterol, hypertension, and inflammation are all metabolic indicators that can significantly increase cardiovascular risks.

4. **Metabolic Syndrome**: This syndrome is a cluster of conditions, including high blood pressure, high blood sugar, excess body fat around the waist, and abnormal cholesterol levels. It increases the risk of heart disease and diabetes and is often linked to poor metabolic health.

5. **Non-Alcoholic Fatty Liver Disease (NAFLD)**: Characterized by fat accumulation in the liver not due to alcohol consumption, NAFLD is associated with

obesity and insulin resistance. It can progress to more severe liver conditions if not addressed.

Understanding these conditions highlights the critical link between metabolism and overall health. By recognizing the underlying metabolic issues, individuals can take proactive steps to mitigate their risks.

How to Prevent Diseases Through Metabolism

Preventing chronic diseases through metabolic health involves adopting a holistic approach focused on lifestyle changes. Here are key strategies to enhance metabolic function and reduce disease risk:

1.   **Balanced Nutrition**: A well-rounded diet rich in whole foods, including fruits, vegetables, lean proteins, and healthy fats, supports metabolic health. Emphasizing nutrient-dense foods helps regulate blood sugar and improve insulin sensitivity. For instance, incorporating fiber-rich foods can stabilize blood sugar levels and promote a healthy gut microbiome.

2.   **Regular Physical Activity**: Exercise plays a vital role in enhancing metabolic health. Engaging in both aerobic exercises, like walking or cycling, and strength training can improve insulin sensitivity, increase energy expenditure, and support weight management. Aiming for at least 150 minutes of moderate-intensity exercise per week can significantly lower the risk of chronic diseases.

3.   **Adequate Sleep**: Sleep is often overlooked in discussions about metabolic health, yet it is crucial for hormone regulation and overall well-being. Poor sleep can disrupt metabolic processes and lead to weight gain and insulin resistance. Prioritizing 7-9 hours of quality sleep per night supports metabolic function and reduces disease risk.

4.   **Stress Management**: Chronic stress can have detrimental effects on metabolic health, primarily through elevated cortisol levels, which can lead to weight gain, particularly around the abdomen. Incorporating stress-reduction techniques such as mindfulness, meditation, or yoga can improve overall health and metabolic balance.

5.   **Regular Monitoring**: Keeping track of key health metrics, such as blood glucose, cholesterol levels, and body composition, allows individuals to identify potential issues early on. Regular check-ups with healthcare providers can help tailor health

strategies to individual needs, making it easier to prevent chronic diseases through proactive metabolic management.

1.4 Case Studies: Success Stories

Health is a deeply personal journey, but learning from others' experiences can offer valuable insights and inspiration. In this section, we'll explore real-life stories of individuals who have transformed their health through lifestyle changes, diet modifications, and perseverance. These case studies highlight not only the tangible results but also the lessons learned from each unique path to wellness.

Real-Life Examples of Health Improvement

One of the most compelling aspects of health journeys is the variety of success stories that demonstrate the power of small, consistent changes.

Take Sarah, a 45-year-old mother of two who had struggled with her weight for most of her adult life. Sarah tried countless diets, from the latest trendy cleanses to extreme calorie restriction, all with little lasting success. Frustrated, she realized she needed to shift her focus from temporary fixes to sustainable, long-term habits. Working with a nutritionist, Sarah adopted a balanced diet that emphasized whole foods, adequate protein, and healthy fats. She incorporated light physical activity into her routine, starting with short daily walks and gradually building up to more intense exercise. Within a year, Sarah had lost 30 pounds, but more importantly, she reported feeling more energized, sleeping better, and noticing significant improvements in her mood. Her journey wasn't without setbacks—holidays and stress occasionally derailed her progress—but Sarah learned to accept that occasional missteps were part of the process, not failures. Her story is a testament to the power of persistence and the importance of creating a plan that fits into one's life, rather than a rigid set of rules that feel like a chore.

In another case, we have John, a 60-year-old man who had been diagnosed with Type 2 diabetes. John was initially overwhelmed by his diagnosis, but with the help of his healthcare provider, he embraced a low-carbohydrate diet and began incorporating intermittent fasting. Unlike many others who feared the restrictions of a lower-carb lifestyle, John found that the flexibility of intermittent fasting allowed him to feel more in control of his eating patterns. Over time, he lost 20 pounds, lowered his blood sugar levels, and was able to reduce his reliance on medication. John's success demonstrates the role of dietary changes in managing chronic conditions, and the empowering effect of reclaiming one's health.

These real-life examples emphasize that health improvements don't happen overnight, but with patience and a personalized approach, it is possible to achieve lasting results. Whether someone's goal is to lose weight, manage a chronic illness, or simply feel better, the keys to success often lie in small, intentional changes and the determination to keep going.

Lessons Learned from Experiences

From these stories, a few recurring lessons stand out. First, sustainability is crucial. Fad diets and extreme regimens often lead to quick results, but they are rarely maintainable in the long term. Sarah and John both found success through gradual changes that were realistic for their daily lives. This highlights the importance of making adjustments that fit into a routine rather than adopting an all-or-nothing mentality.

Second, setbacks are normal. No journey is perfect, and the path to better health will likely involve detours. Both Sarah and John experienced challenges along the way, but their resilience allowed them to stay on course. This is an important reminder for anyone embarking on a health journey: progress isn't linear, but persistence is what ultimately leads to success.

While personal motivation is essential, having a network of support, whether it's from family, healthcare providers, or a community, can make all the difference. Both individuals sought guidance from professionals—Sarah worked with a nutritionist, while John collaborated with his doctor to manage his diabetes. These relationships helped them stay accountable and encouraged them to stay on track even when things got tough. Health improvement is deeply personal and varied. The path that works for one person may not work for another, but the core principles of sustainability, resilience, and support can be applied to any situation. By learning from these case studies, readers can glean valuable insights into how to approach their own wellness journeys with confidence and clarity.

1.5 Tools for Monitoring Health

In today's world, monitoring health has never been easier or more accessible. With advances in technology, we have the ability to track nearly every aspect of our wellbeing, from daily steps and heart rate to sleep patterns and nutrition intake. These tools offer more than just data—they provide insights into our bodies and behaviors, helping us make informed decisions about our health. In this section, we'll explore the most effective technologies, apps, and devices for health monitoring, along with practical tips on how to make the best use of them.

Available Technologies

The rise of wearable technology has revolutionized health monitoring. Devices like fitness trackers, smartwatches, and heart rate monitors have become integral to many people's lives. These gadgets can track daily physical activity, calories burned, and even stress levels. One of the most popular wearables is the smartwatch, which combines multiple health functions in one device. For example, it can monitor heart rate, sleep patterns, and, in some models, even track blood oxygen levels—a crucial metric for anyone with respiratory or cardiovascular concerns.

For those focusing on exercise, wearables can track everything from the number of steps taken each day to more detailed metrics like VO2 max, which measures cardiovascular fitness. These data points allow users to better understand their physical activity levels and make necessary adjustments to improve their overall health. Additionally, heart rate variability, which can be tracked by many wearables, provides insight into how well the body is recovering from exercise or stress, helping individuals avoid burnout or overtraining. In addition to fitness, many people now use continuous glucose monitors (CGMs) to track blood sugar levels in real-time. These devices are especially useful for individuals with diabetes, but they're also gaining popularity among people who want to optimize their nutrition and metabolic health. A CGM can provide immediate feedback on how certain foods affect blood sugar levels, offering valuable insights for those trying to stabilize their energy levels or prevent metabolic conditions.

Useful Apps and Devices

Beyond wearable tech, health monitoring apps have become indispensable tools. These apps serve as personal wellness coaches, helping users stay on top of their health goals. Some of the most popular categories include nutrition tracking, sleep analysis, and mental wellness apps. One such app, MyFitnessPal, allows users to log their meals, track macronutrients, and monitor calorie intake. It's a comprehensive tool that helps people understand what they're consuming on a daily basis and whether they're meeting their nutrition goals. Other apps like Cronometer go even further by breaking down food intake into micronutrients, providing a detailed look at vitamin and mineral consumption. Sleep is another critical aspect of health, and apps like Sleep Cycle have been designed to optimize rest. These apps use sensors to track sleep cycles, offering insights into how long and how well one sleeps. They can also provide suggestions for improving sleep quality, such as adjusting bedtime or room temperature, and even waking users up at the most optimal time during their sleep cycle. For mental health, apps like Headspace and Calm focus on mindfulness and stress reduction, guiding users through meditation exercises that can reduce anxiety and improve mental clarity. These apps are particularly useful for those looking to manage stress, a major factor that affects overall health and metabolic function.

Tips for Effective Use

While technology offers an incredible array of tools to monitor health, knowing how to use these devices and apps effectively is key. The first step is to avoid becoming overwhelmed by the sheer volume of data these tools can provide. It's easy to get caught up in the numbers—whether it's steps, calories, or sleep quality—but the real value lies in understanding trends over time rather than obsessing over day-to-day fluctuations.

For example, instead of focusing on hitting a specific number of steps each day, consider using step data to gauge overall activity levels over the course of a week. If you notice that certain days are less active, you can then plan to incorporate more movement on those days. Similarly, if your sleep app shows that you're consistently getting less rest during the week, you can take steps to improve your sleep hygiene, such as going to bed earlier or creating a more relaxing bedtime routine.

Another important tip is to integrate these tools into a broader wellness plan. Wearable devices and apps are just one piece of the puzzle—they should complement, not replace, other healthy habits. Regular exercise, balanced nutrition, and mental health practices are all crucial to achieving overall wellness. For instance, tracking your nutrition through an app can be a great way to maintain a healthy diet, but it's equally important to ensure that the foods you're choosing align with your personal health goals. Lastly, it's essential to remain consistent. Health monitoring tools are most effective when used regularly. However, consistency doesn't mean perfection. There will be days when you fall short of your goals, but the data collected over time will give you a clearer picture of your overall progress. Use this information to make small, sustainable changes, rather than making drastic shifts that are difficult to maintain.

2. NUTRITION FOR METABOLISM

2.1 Basics of a Balanced Diet

A balanced diet is the cornerstone of metabolic health. It provides the body with the necessary nutrients to maintain energy levels, support bodily functions, and optimize metabolism. Understanding the balance between macronutrients, micronutrients, hydration, and fiber is crucial for anyone aiming to improve their overall health. In this section, we'll explore the fundamental components of a balanced diet, why they are essential for metabolism, and how to avoid common dietary traps that can hinder progress.

Macronutrients and Micronutrients

The foundation of any diet lies in macronutrients: carbohydrates, proteins, and fats. Each macronutrient serves specific roles in the body and has a direct impact on metabolism.

Carbohydrates are the body's primary source of energy, particularly for the brain and muscles. When consumed, carbohydrates break down into glucose, which fuels cellular processes. Complex carbohydrates, found in whole grains, vegetables, and legumes, provide a slower, more sustained release of energy, promoting stable blood sugar levels. In contrast, refined carbs, such as those in white bread and sugary snacks, cause sharp spikes in blood sugar, leading to energy crashes and cravings. The key is to focus on complex carbohydrates that offer fiber and other nutrients, which we'll discuss later in this section.

Proteins play a critical role in building and repairing tissues, producing enzymes and hormones, and supporting immune function. Protein also has a significant thermic effect, meaning it requires more energy to digest compared to carbohydrates and fats. This makes it particularly beneficial for boosting metabolism and maintaining muscle mass. Good sources of protein include lean meats, fish, eggs, dairy, legumes, and plant-based alternatives like tofu or tempeh. A diet rich in protein helps ensure that the body has the raw materials needed to function optimally while also enhancing feelings of satiety, reducing the likelihood of overeating.

Fats are often misunderstood but are equally vital to a balanced diet. Healthy fats, such as those found in olive oil, avocados, nuts, and fatty fish, are essential for brain function, hormone production, and the absorption of fat-soluble vitamins (A, D, E, and K). Fats also provide a long-lasting source of energy, keeping blood sugar stable and preventing energy crashes. It's important to differentiate between healthy unsaturated fats and unhealthy trans fats, which are found in many processed and fried foods. Trans fats can increase the risk of chronic diseases like heart disease and should be minimized as much as possible.

While macronutrients provide the bulk of energy and structural materials, **micronutrients**—vitamins and minerals—play a vital supporting role. They act as cofactors in metabolic processes, supporting everything from immune function to bone health. For example, B-vitamins are essential for converting food into energy, while magnesium is crucial for hundreds of enzymatic reactions in the body. Ensuring a diet rich in fruits, vegetables, and whole foods will help supply a wide range of vitamins and minerals necessary for optimal metabolism.

Importance of Fiber and Hydration

Fiber is a frequently overlooked component of a balanced diet but is indispensable for digestive health and metabolic function. Found in plant-based foods like fruits, vegetables, legumes, and whole grains, fiber comes in two forms: soluble and insoluble.

Soluble fiber, found in foods like oats, apples, and beans, dissolves in water and forms a gel-like substance in the digestive tract. This slows digestion, helping to regulate blood sugar levels and lower cholesterol. For metabolic health, soluble fiber can improve insulin sensitivity and reduce the risk of type 2 diabetes.

Insoluble fiber, present in foods like whole grains, nuts, and vegetables, doesn't dissolve in water and adds bulk to the stool. This type of fiber promotes regular bowel movements, preventing constipation and supporting a healthy gut. Since a healthy digestive system is integral to overall health, ensuring adequate fiber intake is essential for anyone focused on metabolic wellness. In addition to fiber, **hydration** plays a critical role in maintaining metabolism. Water is involved in nearly every bodily function, from regulating body temperature to aiding in digestion and nutrient absorption. Even mild dehydration can slow down metabolic processes and lead to feelings of fatigue. Drinking water also helps with appetite control; sometimes, feelings of hunger are actually a signal for hydration. To stay adequately hydrated, most people should aim for at least eight 8-ounce glasses of water a day, though individual needs may vary based on activity levels, climate, and specific health conditions. Additionally, consuming water-rich foods like fruits and vegetables can contribute to overall hydration. Avoiding excessive intake of caffeinated or sugary drinks is essential, as they can lead to dehydration and disrupt metabolic processes.

Avoiding Dietary Traps

Even with the best intentions, it's easy to fall into common dietary traps that undermine metabolic health. One such trap is **over-restricting calories**. While reducing calorie intake can lead to weight loss, severe calorie restriction can slow metabolism as the body enters "starvation mode." This adaptive response conserves energy, making it harder to lose weight and maintain energy levels. Instead of drastic cuts, focus on creating a modest calorie deficit, if needed, while ensuring adequate nutrient intake.

Another trap is **relying on processed "diet" foods**. Many products marketed as low-fat or low-carb are often highly processed and filled with artificial ingredients, preservatives, or added sugars. These products may offer fewer calories or fat grams, but they often lack the nutrients found in whole, unprocessed foods. They can also disrupt metabolism by causing blood sugar spikes or triggering cravings. It's far better to focus on whole, minimally processed foods that provide lasting energy and essential nutrients.

Finally, beware of **neglecting nutrient diversity**. Many people get stuck in a dietary rut, eating the same foods day after day. While consistency can be helpful, a lack of variety can lead to nutrient deficiencies, which may hinder metabolic processes. Incorporating a range of foods—especially different colored fruits and vegetables—ensures a broader spectrum of vitamins, minerals, and phytonutrients that support overall health.

2.2 Dietary Philosophies: Which to Choose?

Navigating the world of dietary philosophies can be overwhelming, especially with the abundance of approaches available today. From the all-meat **Carnivore** diet to the plant-based **Vegan** diet, people often find themselves drawn to specific philosophies for various health, ethical, or personal reasons. In this section, we'll examine several prominent dietary approaches, outline their potential benefits and drawbacks, and explore universal dietary principles that can benefit anyone, regardless of the specific diet they follow.

Carnivore, Vegan, and Beyond

There is no one-size-fits-all when it comes to diet, and the variety of approaches reflects this. Below are some of the most popular dietary philosophies:

Carnivore Diet: This diet focuses almost exclusively on animal products like meat, fish, eggs, and certain dairy products, excluding plant-based foods entirely. Proponents claim it can help with weight loss, inflammation reduction, and mental clarity. By eliminating carbohydrates and fiber, the Carnivore diet forces the body to rely on fats for energy, potentially putting individuals in a state of ketosis.

Benefits: The Carnivore diet is highly satiating, making it easier for some people to control hunger and caloric intake. For individuals with certain autoimmune conditions, removing plant-based irritants might help alleviate symptoms.

Drawbacks: This diet lacks fiber and essential vitamins found in plant-based foods, such as vitamin C and antioxidants. Over time, this can lead to nutrient deficiencies and potential digestive issues. Additionally, the long-term effects of an all-meat diet on heart health remain controversial.

Vegan Diet: In contrast to Carnivore, the Vegan diet excludes all animal products, focusing on fruits, vegetables, legumes, grains, nuts, and seeds. Vegans avoid meat, dairy, eggs, and honey, primarily for ethical, environmental, or health reasons.

Benefits: A well-planned Vegan diet can be rich in vitamins, minerals, antioxidants, and fiber, supporting heart health, weight management, and improved digestion. Studies have shown that plant-based diets may lower the risk of chronic diseases such as diabetes, heart disease, and certain cancers.

Drawbacks: Vegans must be diligent in ensuring they get enough protein, iron, calcium, vitamin B12, and omega-3 fatty acids, as these nutrients are primarily found in animal products. Without careful planning or supplementation, nutrient deficiencies may arise. Some individuals also find it difficult to maintain muscle mass on a strictly plant-based diet.

Mediterranean Diet: This diet emphasizes whole grains, fruits, vegetables, lean proteins (especially fish), and healthy fats like olive oil. Inspired by the traditional eating habits of countries bordering the Mediterranean Sea, it's considered one of the most balanced and sustainable diets.

Benefits: The Mediterranean diet is rich in antioxidants, healthy fats, fiber, and lean proteins, supporting heart health, cognitive function, and longevity. It's also relatively easy to maintain long-term, with a variety of flavorful foods.

Drawbacks: For those with dietary restrictions or specific health goals (such as rapid weight loss), the Mediterranean diet might not provide fast results. Additionally, the inclusion of grains and moderate amounts of alcohol (wine) may not suit everyone's preferences or health needs.

Paleo Diet: The Paleo diet seeks to mimic the eating habits of our hunter-gatherer ancestors, focusing on unprocessed foods like meats, fish, vegetables, fruits, nuts, and seeds, while excluding grains, legumes, and dairy. The premise is that these foods are more natural for human consumption and better support health.

Benefits: By eliminating processed foods and sugars, the Paleo diet can improve energy levels, digestion, and weight management. It's also rich in protein and fiber, supporting muscle mass and gut health.

Drawbacks: Excluding entire food groups (grains, legumes, and dairy) can make it challenging to meet daily nutrient needs. This may lead to nutrient deficiencies over time if the diet is not carefully balanced.

Benefits and Drawbacks of Different Diets

When choosing a dietary philosophy, it's essential to weigh both the benefits and drawbacks, as different approaches will suit different lifestyles, health goals, and individual needs.

Benefits of Specific Diets:

●**Carnivore**: Simplicity, hunger control, and possible autoimmune benefits.

●**Vegan**: Ethical considerations, environmental sustainability, and chronic disease prevention.

●**Mediterranean**: Balanced, heart-healthy, and easy to maintain.

●**Paleo**: Focus on unprocessed foods, energy, and digestive benefits.

However, each diet comes with potential drawbacks:

●**Carnivore**: Lacks plant-based nutrients, risk of nutrient deficiencies.

●**Vegan**: Requires careful planning to avoid deficiencies, can be challenging to maintain muscle mass.

●**Mediterranean**: May not deliver fast results or suit specific health goals.

●**Paleo**: Restrictive, excluding major food groups, which may lead to nutrient imbalances.

Ultimately, the choice of diet should align with an individual's health goals, ethical beliefs, and personal preferences. No one diet works for everyone, and the key is finding an approach that feels sustainable, enjoyable, and nourishing.

Universal Dietary Principles

Regardless of the diet you choose, there are universal principles that can help guide your eating habits to promote long-term health and support metabolism:

1.   **Focus on Whole Foods**: Whole, unprocessed foods should make up the bulk of any diet. These foods are nutrient-dense, high in vitamins and minerals, and free from artificial additives. Whether it's fresh vegetables, lean proteins, or healthy fats, whole foods are always a better choice than processed alternatives.

2.   **Moderation is Key**: Even with healthy diets, moderation is essential. Overeating, even nutrient-dense foods, can lead to weight gain and metabolic disruptions. Listening to your body's hunger cues and avoiding extremes—whether overeating or undereating—will help maintain balance.

3.   **Stay Hydrated**: Water is critical to maintaining a healthy metabolism, regardless of the dietary philosophy you follow. Drinking enough water helps digestion,

nutrient absorption, and energy production. Aim to drink water consistently throughout the day, and consider water-rich foods to support hydration.

4.   **Variety is Vital**: Eating a wide variety of foods ensures that you're getting a full range of nutrients. Don't rely too heavily on one food group or type of food. By incorporating different sources of proteins, fats, and carbohydrates, along with various fruits and vegetables, you'll provide your body with everything it needs to function optimally.

5.   **Avoid Processed Foods**: Highly processed foods are often loaded with added sugars, unhealthy fats, and preservatives. They can disrupt blood sugar levels, promote weight gain, and cause inflammation. No matter what dietary philosophy you choose, minimizing processed foods is key to supporting metabolic health and longevity.

2.3 Recipes for Metabolic Wellness

Maintaining a healthy metabolism is a dynamic process, deeply connected to what we eat and how we nourish our bodies throughout the day. Metabolism isn't just about burning calories; it's a comprehensive system that regulates everything from energy production to the way our body stores fat and maintains muscle mass. To support optimal metabolic function, our meals must be nutrient-dense, well-balanced, and tailored to our unique needs. This section explores how to create meals that not only taste great but also fuel your body effectively.

Balanced and Nutrient-Dense Meals

A well-balanced meal is one that provides a harmonious blend of macronutrients and micronutrients, without tipping the scales too far in any one direction. While it's easy to get lost in trends or restrictive diets, the foundation of good nutrition is balance. For example, take a classic grilled chicken dish served with a side of sautéed spinach and roasted sweet potatoes. At first glance, this meal might seem simple, but it's an excellent example of nutrient balance. The grilled chicken provides lean protein, essential for muscle repair and overall metabolism. The spinach offers fiber, vitamins A and C, and iron, all of which are crucial for cellular functions. Sweet potatoes add complex carbohydrates, which release energy gradually, supporting sustained activity without spiking blood sugar levels. These types of meals are crucial for keeping your metabolism in check. When your diet is based on nutrient-dense foods, you're providing your body with the fuel it needs to perform its daily functions optimally. Protein helps maintain muscle mass, which is essential for a strong metabolism. Carbohydrates fuel your brain and body, but choosing slow-digesting options like whole grains and vegetables prevents crashes in energy levels. Fats, especially those found in nuts, seeds, and oils like olive oil, are equally important, as they support hormone balance and the absorption of fat-soluble vitamins.

On the flip side, meals that lack variety or rely too heavily on processed foods can slow your metabolism. Over time, nutrient deficiencies build up, your energy wanes, and your body starts to struggle with basic metabolic processes. It's not about rigidly following a particular diet, but rather, about listening to your body and incorporating a wide array of whole foods into your daily routine.

Another example of a balanced meal might be a colorful quinoa salad with grilled salmon, avocado, and a lemon-tahini dressing. This dish incorporates healthy fats from the avocado and salmon, which are rich in omega-3s, known to reduce inflammation and support heart health. The quinoa provides plant-based protein and fiber, while the lemon-tahini dressing adds flavor without overloading the dish with unnecessary calories. Each ingredient works synergistically, contributing to overall metabolic wellness by ensuring your body has the right tools to function at its best.

Healthy Snacks for the Day

Snacks are often where our best intentions can go awry. When hunger strikes mid-morning or late afternoon, it's all too easy to reach for whatever's most convenient, whether it's a sugary granola bar or a bag of chips. But the choices we make between meals are just as important as the meals themselves. Snacking doesn't have to derail your metabolic health; in fact, the right snacks can help stabilize blood sugar, keep hunger at bay, and ensure that you have sustained energy throughout the day. The key is choosing snacks that are rich in protein, fiber, and healthy fats—while steering clear of those that are high in sugar and refined carbs. One snack that works well for metabolism is a small handful of mixed nuts paired with a piece of fruit. The nuts provide a good source of fat and protein, which help to stabilize blood sugar and prevent energy dips, while the fruit offers natural sugars and fiber, making it a well-rounded option. Another excellent choice is Greek yogurt with a sprinkling of chia seeds or flaxseeds. Yogurt is a great source of protein and probiotics, which can aid digestion and support gut health—a critical factor in metabolism. The seeds provide fiber and omega-3s, adding both texture and nutritional benefits to your snack.

For those who prefer something more savory, a small serving of hummus with raw vegetables can be an ideal option. The hummus offers plant-based protein and fiber from the chickpeas, while the vegetables, like carrots and cucumbers, are low in calories but high in water and fiber, promoting fullness without weighing you down. Alternatively, a boiled egg paired with a slice of avocado can be a quick snack that packs in both protein and healthy fats, helping you stay satiated until your next meal. It's important to keep in mind that portion control is key when it comes to snacking. Even healthy snacks can become problematic if consumed in excess, as too many calories can lead to weight gain, which in turn slows your metabolism. The goal is to fuel your body between meals in a way that supports energy levels and prevents overeating when it's time for your next full meal.

Meal Planning Tips

Planning meals in advance is one of the most effective strategies for maintaining metabolic wellness. When you plan ahead, you're less likely to make impulsive food choices that could derail your progress. Instead, you can focus on creating balanced, nutrient-dense meals that fit your specific needs and goals. Start by setting aside time each week to plan your meals and snacks. Consider your schedule: if you know you'll have a particularly busy day, plan for quick, easy meals that don't require much prep work, like a salad with pre-grilled chicken or a smoothie loaded with greens, protein powder, and healthy fats like almond butter. Planning in this way ensures that even when life gets hectic, you're still nourishing your body in a way that supports your metabolism. When meal prepping, focus on building a variety of meals that incorporate different flavors, textures, and nutrients. Batch cooking is a great way to stay on track throughout the week. For instance, roasting a large tray of vegetables on Sunday can serve as the foundation for multiple meals—add them to quinoa for lunch one day and pair them with grilled chicken for dinner another day. Similarly, preparing a large batch of protein, like chicken or salmon, can make it easier to throw together healthy meals when time is short. In addition to meal prepping, it's helpful to keep your pantry stocked with go-to ingredients that can be turned into quick, nutritious meals. Items like canned beans, lentils, whole grains, olive oil, and frozen vegetables are great staples to have on hand. When your kitchen is stocked with healthy options, it becomes easier to avoid processed or less nutritious foods.

Finally, don't forget to keep hydration top of mind. Drinking water throughout the day is just as important as the food you eat when it comes to metabolic health. Water helps your body process nutrients, supports digestion, and keeps your energy levels stable. Aim to drink water regularly throughout the day and incorporate water-rich foods like cucumbers, watermelon, and leafy greens into your meals.

Meal planning doesn't have to be time-consuming or complex. By taking small, consistent steps each week, you can create an eating plan that supports your metabolism, fuels your body, and makes healthy eating a habit.

2.4 The Importance of Intermittent Fasting

Intermittent fasting (IF) has become increasingly popular as a method for improving metabolic health and overall well-being. While it may seem like just another trend, fasting has been practiced for centuries in various cultures for spiritual, mental, and physical reasons. Modern science supports the benefits of intermittent fasting, showing that it can help regulate blood sugar levels, promote fat loss, enhance mental clarity, and even extend lifespan. But as with any health practice, it's essential to understand the underlying principles and how to implement it safely.

Benefits and Methods

At its core, intermittent fasting isn't about what you eat, but rather when you eat. The idea is to create specific windows of time during which you consume your meals, followed by extended periods of fasting. The fasting periods allow your body to enter a state where it burns stored fat for energy, a process called lipolysis, and becomes more efficient in using nutrients. The benefits of intermittent fasting go beyond just weight management.

One of the main advantages is improved insulin sensitivity. Insulin is a hormone responsible for regulating blood sugar levels, and when your body becomes resistant to it, you're at a higher risk of developing type 2 diabetes. Intermittent fasting helps lower insulin levels, allowing your body to use stored glucose more effectively and reducing the risk of insulin resistance. Another significant benefit is autophagy, a natural process in which the body clears out damaged cells and regenerates new, healthy ones. Autophagy is particularly beneficial for longevity and reducing the risk of diseases such as cancer and Alzheimer's. Fasting triggers this cellular repair process, giving your body the time and space to heal itself. There are several methods of intermittent fasting, each with its own unique approach. One of the most popular is the 16:8 method, where you fast for 16 hours and eat all your meals within an 8-hour window. For example, you might choose to eat only between noon and 8 PM, allowing your body to fast overnight and into the morning. This method is relatively easy to follow, as much of the fasting period occurs while you're sleeping.

Another common method is the 5:2 plan, where you eat normally for five days of the week and significantly reduce your calorie intake (to around 500–600 calories) for the remaining two days. This approach allows for more flexibility, as you're only restricting your intake a couple of days per week while still reaping the metabolic benefits of fasting.

The Eat-Stop-Eat method is a more intensive form of intermittent fasting, where you fast for a full 24 hours once or twice a week. While this method can be effective for some, it requires a bit more discipline and isn't recommended for beginners. There's the alternate-day fasting method, which involves fasting every other day. On fasting days, you either don't eat or drastically reduce your calorie intake, while on non-fasting days, you eat normally. This method can lead to significant fat loss but might be too restrictive for some people to maintain in the long term.

How to Implement It Safely

While intermittent fasting can offer numerous benefits, it's important to approach it with caution, especially if you're new to fasting or have any pre-existing health conditions. First and foremost, it's crucial to listen to your body. If fasting leaves you feeling overly fatigued, irritable, or lightheaded, it may not be the right approach for you—or you might need to adjust your fasting schedule to make it more manageable.

One of the key factors in safely practicing intermittent fasting is staying hydrated. Since you'll be going without food for extended periods, drinking enough water is essential to prevent dehydration, which can exacerbate feelings of hunger and fatigue. You can also consume non-caloric beverages like herbal tea or black coffee during fasting periods to help keep your energy levels stable.

Another important consideration is the quality of the food you eat during your eating window. While intermittent fasting can help control calorie intake, it doesn't give you a free pass to indulge in unhealthy foods. Focus on nutrient-dense, whole foods that provide sustained energy and support overall metabolic health. Think of it this way: fasting gives your body the chance to "clean house," and you want to fill it back up with high-quality nutrients, not junk food that will undo the benefits of fasting. If you're concerned about how fasting might affect your energy levels, especially when it comes to exercising, it's helpful to experiment with different workout timings. Some people prefer to work out during their fasting period, as this can help boost fat burning. Others find that they have more energy and perform better if they eat a small, nutrient-dense meal beforehand. Again, this comes down to listening to your body and finding what works best for you. Intermittent fasting isn't recommended for everyone. If you have a history of eating disorders, are pregnant, breastfeeding, or managing certain health conditions, it's best to consult with a healthcare professional before beginning any fasting regimen. Fasting can also affect hormone levels, particularly in women, so it's important to proceed carefully and ensure that your fasting plan aligns with your body's needs.

Sample Fasting Plans

For those new to intermittent fasting, starting with a gradual approach can help ease the transition. Below are a few sample fasting plans to give you an idea of how to structure your fasting and eating windows:

1.   **16:8 Plan**
Fasting window: 8 PM to 12 PM (16 hours)
Eating window: 12 PM to 8 PM (8 hours)
In this plan, you skip breakfast and focus on having two or three balanced meals during the eating window. For example, you could have a salad with grilled chicken for lunch, a

handful of nuts for an afternoon snack, and a balanced dinner of salmon, quinoa, and steamed vegetables.

2. 5:2 Plan

Regular eating days: Monday, Wednesday, Friday, Saturday, Sunday

Reduced-calorie days: Tuesday, Thursday (500–600 calories)

On the two fasting days, you might have a light breakfast, such as scrambled eggs with spinach, and a simple dinner of vegetable soup. The rest of the week, you eat normally while still focusing on whole, nutrient-dense foods.

3. Eat-Stop-Eat Plan

Fast once or twice a week for 24 hours

On fasting days, you would go from dinner one day until dinner the next, consuming only water, tea, or coffee during the fasting period. After the 24-hour fast, resume eating a balanced, nutrient-dense meal.

4. Alternate-Day Fasting Plan

Monday, Wednesday, Friday: Fasting days (500–600 calories)

Tuesday, Thursday, Saturday, Sunday: Regular eating days

On fasting days, you might stick to a small meal like a vegetable stir-fry or a smoothie with protein powder and greens. On regular days, focus on balanced meals that provide a good mix of proteins, healthy fats, and complex carbs.

These plans can be adjusted based on your personal preferences and lifestyle. The key is to find a schedule that works for you and supports your long-term health goals. Remember, intermittent fasting is not a one-size-fits-all solution, but rather a tool that can be tailored to your unique needs.

2.5 Foods that Support Health

Food is more than fuel; it's a critical component of your overall health and well-being. What you put into your body has a direct impact on your metabolism, immune system, and even your mental health. By making conscious choices about the foods you eat, you can influence inflammation, enhance your energy levels, and boost your body's ability to manage stress. This section explores the powerful effects of anti-inflammatory foods, the role of superfoods in metabolic health, and how to make intentional food choices that promote lasting well-being.

Anti-Inflammatory Foods

Chronic inflammation is at the root of many modern diseases, from heart disease and diabetes to arthritis and even certain cancers. Inflammation itself isn't inherently harmful—it's a natural response that your body uses to fight off infections and heal injuries. However, when it becomes chronic, it can lead to a variety of health issues, silently damaging tissues and organs over time. The good news is that you can control much of the inflammation in your body through the foods you eat. A diet rich in anti-inflammatory foods can act as a protective shield against the detrimental effects of chronic inflammation. Anti-inflammatory foods are those that help reduce or prevent the inflammatory response in the body. These include foods rich in omega-3 fatty acids, antioxidants, and polyphenols. Omega-3 fatty acids, which are commonly found in fatty fish like salmon and sardines, work to balance out the inflammatory effects of omega-6 fatty acids, which are often abundant in processed and fried foods. Inflammation occurs when there's an imbalance between omega-6 and omega-3 levels, and consuming more omega-3s helps bring that balance back in check.

Antioxidants play a crucial role in fighting inflammation by neutralizing free radicals, which are unstable molecules that cause cellular damage. Berries such as blueberries, strawberries, and raspberries are packed with antioxidants, particularly a type called flavonoids, which have been shown to reduce the markers of inflammation in the body. Flavonoids are also abundant in other plant-based foods like green tea, dark chocolate, and citrus fruits. Leafy greens, such as spinach, kale, and Swiss chard, are another powerful weapon in the fight against inflammation. They're high in vitamins A, C, and K, as well as minerals like magnesium, which have anti-inflammatory properties. Vitamin K, in particular, is critical in reducing inflammatory markers and has been associated with a decreased risk of conditions like osteoporosis and arthritis. Another potent anti-inflammatory food group is spices, with turmeric standing out as one of the most studied and beneficial. Turmeric contains curcumin, a compound known for its powerful anti-inflammatory effects. It's been shown to block molecules in the body that trigger inflammation, making it effective for managing conditions like arthritis and inflammatory bowel disease. Ginger is another spice with similar benefits, often used to reduce nausea, improve digestion, and decrease inflammation in the muscles after intense physical activity. Olive oil, especially extra virgin olive oil, is another cornerstone of an anti-inflammatory diet. It's rich in monounsaturated fats and contains oleocanthal, a compound that has been shown to reduce inflammation similarly to ibuprofen. In Mediterranean cultures, olive oil is a staple, and it's no coincidence that these populations often have lower rates of inflammatory diseases. While it's important to focus on anti-inflammatory foods, it's equally crucial to avoid foods that contribute to inflammation. Processed sugars, refined carbohydrates, and trans fats are some of the biggest offenders. These foods not only increase inflammation but also contribute to weight gain, which is a major risk factor for inflammatory diseases. Instead, choosing whole, unprocessed foods that are rich in nutrients helps keep inflammation at bay and supports overall health.

Superfoods for Metabolic Health

The term "superfoods" has gained popularity over the years, but it's not just a marketing gimmick. Superfoods are nutrient-dense, providing high amounts of vitamins, minerals, antioxidants, and other compounds that are essential for good health. While no single food can fix all of your health problems, incorporating superfoods into your diet can significantly enhance your metabolic function and overall well-being.

Metabolism is the process by which your body converts what you eat and drink into energy. A healthy metabolism ensures that your body efficiently uses the nutrients you consume, helping you maintain a healthy weight, improve energy levels, and reduce the risk of metabolic disorders like type 2 diabetes. Certain superfoods have been shown to specifically support metabolic health by boosting your body's ability to burn fat, regulate blood sugar, and manage energy. One of the top superfoods for metabolism is green tea. It contains a powerful antioxidant called epigallocatechin gallate (EGCG), which has been shown to increase fat burning and improve metabolic rate. In addition to EGCG, green tea contains caffeine, which can further enhance metabolic function by increasing thermogenesis—the process by which your body generates heat and burns calories. Studies suggest that regular consumption of green tea can lead to modest weight loss and improvements in body composition. Another superfood that supports metabolic health is chia seeds. These tiny seeds are packed with fiber, which slows the absorption of carbohydrates and helps regulate blood sugar levels. They're also rich in omega-3 fatty acids and protein, making them a great addition to smoothies, yogurt, or oatmeal. The fiber content in chia seeds promotes a feeling of fullness, helping to reduce overall calorie intake and support weight management. Avocados are often considered a superfood due to their high content of healthy fats, fiber, and a variety of essential nutrients like potassium and magnesium. The monounsaturated fats in avocados help to stabilize blood sugar levels, while the fiber content aids in digestion and keeps you feeling satisfied longer. Potassium plays a key role in maintaining metabolic health by regulating fluid balance, nerve signals, and muscle contractions, all of which are vital for energy production. Berries, particularly blueberries, stand out as metabolic powerhouses. Not only are they rich in antioxidants, but they also contain anthocyanins, which have been shown to improve insulin sensitivity and reduce fat accumulation. The low glycemic index of berries means they won't cause sharp spikes in blood sugar, making them an excellent choice for anyone looking to manage their weight or prevent metabolic syndrome. Greek yogurt is another fantastic superfood for metabolic health. It's high in protein, which helps build and maintain muscle mass—a key component of a healthy metabolism. The probiotics in yogurt support gut health, which plays a significant role in overall metabolism and digestion. A healthy gut microbiome can improve the absorption of nutrients and aid in the regulation of appetite hormones like ghrelin and leptin. Nuts, particularly almonds and walnuts, are nutrient-dense and high in healthy fats, fiber, and protein. Almonds, for instance, are rich in magnesium, which plays a critical role in over 300 metabolic reactions in the body. Walnuts are an excellent source of alpha-linolenic acid (ALA), a plant-based omega-3 fatty acid that can reduce inflammation and improve heart health. Dark chocolate, especially varieties with a high cacao content, is also a surprising but effective superfood for metabolic health. It contains flavonoids that improve insulin sensitivity, reduce inflammation, and support cardiovascular health. Of course, it's important to consume dark chocolate in moderation due to its calorie content, but small amounts can offer significant health benefits.

Making Conscious Food Choices

When it comes to supporting your health through diet, making conscious food choices is key. This involves not just focusing on what you eat, but also understanding where your food comes from, how it's prepared, and how it fits into your overall lifestyle. Conscious eating isn't about adhering to strict dietary rules, but rather about being mindful of the foods you consume and how they affect your body. One of the first steps in making conscious food choices is to prioritize whole, unprocessed foods. These foods are closer to their natural state and are often richer in nutrients compared to processed foods, which are stripped of essential vitamins and minerals. For example, choosing whole grains like quinoa or brown rice over refined grains like white bread or pasta ensures that you're getting more fiber, vitamins, and antioxidants. Similarly, opting for fresh fruits and vegetables over canned or processed varieties means you're consuming more of the nutrients that promote good health. Another aspect of conscious eating is considering the environmental and ethical impact of your food choices. Locally sourced, organic foods often have a lower environmental footprint compared to conventionally grown or imported foods. Organic farming practices also reduce the use of harmful pesticides and support soil health, which in turn leads to more nutrient-dense crops. While organic foods may be more expensive, the long-term benefits for both your health and the environment can outweigh the cost. Portion control is another essential element of making conscious food choices. In today's society, where oversized portions are the norm, it's easy to consume more calories than your body needs. By paying attention to portion sizes and eating mindfully, you can better regulate your calorie intake and avoid the pitfalls of overeating. This doesn't mean you have to meticulously measure everything you eat, but being aware of hunger cues and eating until you're satisfied—not stuffed—can go a long way in maintaining a healthy metabolism. Finally, making conscious food choices involves being aware of how different foods affect your body. Some people may thrive on a plant-based diet, while others may find that they need more animal-based proteins to feel their best. Listening to your body's signals, such as how certain foods make you feel physically and mentally, is crucial in creating a diet that works for you. Everyone's nutritional needs are different, and there's no one-size-fits-all approach when it comes to diet.

Chapter 3: The Role of Sleep and Rest

3.1 Sleep Cycles and Metabolism

Sleep is often viewed as a passive state of rest, but in reality, it's an active and essential process that directly influences nearly every aspect of your health, including metabolism. While you sleep, your body undergoes critical physiological processes that help restore energy, repair tissues, and regulate hormones. Sleep cycles, which consist of various stages, play a significant role in these functions, especially when it comes to metabolism and overall health. In this section, we'll explore how different stages of sleep impact metabolic processes and offer practical techniques for improving sleep quality.

Stages of Sleep

To understand how sleep affects metabolism, it's important to first examine the structure of sleep itself. Sleep isn't a uniform experience but is divided into distinct stages, each playing a unique role in the restoration and recovery of the body and brain. Broadly speaking, sleep is divided into two main categories: rapid eye movement (REM) sleep and non-rapid eye movement (NREM) sleep. Within NREM sleep, there are three stages that progressively deepen.

The first stage of sleep is the transition between wakefulness and sleep, often referred to as light sleep. This is when your body begins to relax, your heart rate and breathing start to slow, and your brain produces theta waves, which are slower in frequency than when you're awake. This stage typically lasts only a few minutes, and while it's the lightest stage of sleep, it's essential for moving into the deeper stages where restorative processes take place.

The second stage of sleep, still considered light sleep, lasts for longer periods and is characterized by further decreases in body temperature, heart rate, and breathing. During this stage, your body becomes more detached from the external environment, preparing for the deeper stages of sleep that follow. Brain activity slows down even more, but there are short bursts of activity called sleep spindles, which are believed to play a role in memory consolidation.

The third stage of NREM sleep is deep sleep, sometimes called slow-wave sleep because of the slow, high-amplitude delta waves that dominate brain activity. This is the most restorative stage of sleep, during which your body does most of its repair work. Growth hormone is released during deep sleep, which is vital for cell regeneration, muscle repair, and overall physical recovery. Additionally, deep sleep is when your immune system is most active, helping to fight off infections and maintain overall health.

Finally, REM sleep is the stage most commonly associated with dreaming. It's during this phase that your brain becomes highly active, processing emotions, experiences, and memories from the day. REM sleep is also crucial for cognitive function, creativity, and emotional regulation. Although your brain is highly active during REM, your body is mostly paralyzed, a mechanism designed to prevent you from physically acting out your dreams.

Each night, you cycle through these stages multiple times, with the majority of deep sleep occurring in the first half of the night and more REM sleep taking place in the early morning hours. These cycles are typically 90 minutes long, and a healthy adult will go through four to six cycles per night. However, the quality and duration of each stage can be influenced by various factors, including stress, diet, lifestyle, and environmental conditions.

Impact of Sleep on Metabolic Health

Sleep is a time of restoration not just for the brain but for the entire body, particularly the metabolic system. During sleep, the body regulates several key hormones involved in metabolism, including insulin, leptin, and cortisol. These hormones play critical roles in hunger, satiety, and the storage and usage of energy.

Insulin, which is responsible for regulating blood sugar levels, becomes less effective when you're sleep-deprived. Research has shown that even just a few nights of poor sleep can lead to insulin resistance, a condition where cells become less responsive to insulin and are unable to efficiently use glucose for energy. This can cause blood sugar levels to rise, increasing the risk of developing type 2 diabetes. Insulin resistance is also linked to weight gain, particularly around the abdomen, which further exacerbates metabolic problems.

Leptin and ghrelin are two hormones that regulate hunger and satiety. Leptin signals to your brain that you're full and should stop eating, while ghrelin stimulates hunger and encourages eating. When you don't get enough sleep, leptin levels drop, and ghrelin levels rise, creating a double-edged sword: you feel hungrier and less satisfied after eating. This hormonal imbalance often leads to overeating, cravings for high-calorie foods, and weight gain.

Cortisol, the stress hormone, also plays a significant role in sleep and metabolism. Cortisol levels should naturally decrease at night, allowing your body to relax and prepare for sleep. However, when you're sleep-deprived or stressed, cortisol levels remain elevated, leading to increased appetite and a tendency to store fat, especially in the abdominal area. Chronic high levels of cortisol can contribute to a slower metabolism, making it harder to lose weight and maintain a healthy body composition.

In addition to hormone regulation, sleep is critical for maintaining proper energy balance. When you're sleep-deprived, your body's ability to process carbohydrates is impaired, leading to higher blood sugar levels and decreased insulin sensitivity. This can result in a cycle of fatigue, overeating, and poor food choices, further disrupting your metabolism. On the flip side, adequate sleep allows your body to metabolize food more efficiently, providing the energy you need to maintain an active lifestyle.

Sleep also affects your basal metabolic rate (BMR), which is the amount of energy your body uses at rest to perform essential functions like breathing, circulation, and temperature regulation. Studies have shown that sleep deprivation can lower your BMR, meaning your body burns fewer calories while at rest. Over time, this can contribute to weight gain and other metabolic issues. Sleep is crucial for physical recovery, especially if you engage in regular exercise. During deep sleep, your body repairs muscle tissue and replenishes energy stores, which is essential for maintaining muscle mass and metabolic health. When you don't get enough deep sleep, your body's ability to recover from physical activity is compromised, leading to fatigue, reduced performance, and a slower metabolism.

Techniques to Improve Sleep Quality

Given the profound impact that sleep has on metabolism and overall health, it's essential to prioritize good sleep hygiene. Improving sleep quality isn't just about getting more hours of rest; it's about optimizing the conditions that allow for restorative sleep cycles. Fortunately, there are several techniques you can implement to enhance your sleep quality and, in turn, support your metabolic health.

One of the most effective ways to improve sleep quality is by establishing a consistent sleep schedule. Going to bed and waking up at the same time every day helps regulate your body's internal clock, also known as the circadian rhythm. Your circadian rhythm controls your sleep-wake cycle, as well as many other bodily functions like hormone production and metabolism. When your sleep schedule is irregular, it can throw off this natural rhythm, making it harder to fall asleep and stay asleep. By sticking to a consistent sleep schedule, even on weekends, you can help reset your circadian rhythm and improve your sleep quality. Creating a relaxing bedtime routine can also signal to your body that it's time to wind down for the night. This could include activities like reading, taking a warm bath, or practicing relaxation techniques such as deep breathing or meditation. The goal is to create a sense of calm and relaxation, allowing your body and mind to transition smoothly from wakefulness to sleep. The sleep environment is another critical factor in sleep quality. Your bedroom should be a quiet, dark, and cool space that promotes relaxation. Exposure to light, especially blue light from screens, can interfere with the production of melatonin, a hormone that regulates sleep. To improve your sleep environment, consider using blackout curtains to block out light, keeping your bedroom at a comfortable temperature (around 60-67°F), and using earplugs or white noise machines to drown out disruptive sounds. Limiting caffeine and alcohol intake is also crucial for improving sleep quality. Caffeine, found in coffee, tea, and some sodas, is a stimulant that can interfere with your ability to fall asleep and stay asleep. Even if you don't feel the effects of caffeine, it can remain in your system for several hours, disrupting your sleep cycles. Similarly, while alcohol may make you feel drowsy initially, it can interfere with REM sleep, leaving you feeling tired and unrested the next day. Exercise is another powerful tool for improving sleep quality, but it's important to time your workouts appropriately. Engaging in regular physical activity can help regulate your sleep-wake cycle, reduce stress, and promote deeper sleep. However, exercising too close to bedtime can have the opposite effect, as it raises your body temperature and stimulates the release of adrenaline. For optimal sleep, aim to finish your workout at least a few hours before bed. Lastly, mindfulness and stress management can play a significant role in improving sleep quality. Stress is one of the leading causes of sleep disturbances, as it triggers the release of cortisol and other stress hormones that make it harder to relax and fall asleep. Incorporating mindfulness practices, such as meditation or progressive muscle relaxation, can help reduce stress and promote a sense of calm before bed.

3.2 Circadian Rhythm and Health

Your circadian rhythm is a 24-hour internal clock that runs in the background of your brain, controlling your sleep-wake cycle and many other vital bodily functions. This rhythm is influenced by external cues like light and temperature, but it's deeply ingrained in your biology, aligning with the natural cycles of day and night. The circadian rhythm doesn't just affect when you feel sleepy or alert—it also has a profound impact on your metabolism, digestion, hormone production, and even your cognitive abilities. Understanding this rhythm can help you make better choices for your diet, exercise, and overall health. In this section, we'll dive into how circadian rhythms work, their implications for your health, and practical strategies for aligning your lifestyle with your natural biological clock.

Understanding Circadian Rhythms

The term "circadian" comes from the Latin words "circa" (meaning around) and "diem" (meaning day), which literally means "about a day." This biological clock is governed by a group of neurons in the hypothalamus known as the suprachiasmatic nucleus (SCN). The SCN responds to light signals received through the eyes and communicates with various systems in the body to regulate functions like sleep, body temperature, digestion, and hormone release. The circadian rhythm operates in cycles that are generally in sync with the 24-hour day, although each person's internal clock may differ slightly. Light is the primary signal that keeps this rhythm in check, but other factors such as meal timing, physical activity, and social interactions also play a role in maintaining its regularity. Disruptions to your circadian rhythm, such as staying up late, working night shifts, or experiencing jet lag, can lead to a host of problems, including sleep disorders, metabolic dysfunction, and cognitive decline. Modern lifestyles, filled with artificial light and irregular schedules, have led many people to fall out of sync with their natural rhythms, contributing to poor health outcomes. By understanding your circadian rhythm and making small adjustments to your daily routine, you can support your body's natural functions and optimize your health. Your circadian rhythm doesn't just influence sleep; it plays a key role in regulating hormone production. Hormones like melatonin, which helps you sleep, and cortisol, which helps you wake up, follow a circadian pattern. Cortisol levels peak in the morning, giving you a burst of energy to start your day, and gradually decrease throughout the day. Melatonin, on the other hand, increases in the evening, preparing your body for rest. In addition to sleep and hormone regulation, circadian rhythms influence your metabolism. Research shows that the timing of meals can impact how efficiently your body processes food. Eating at odd hours or late at night, when your metabolism naturally slows down, can lead to weight gain and metabolic disorders. Aligning your eating habits with your circadian rhythm can help support better digestion, energy balance, and overall metabolic health.

Implications for Diet and Exercise

The connection between circadian rhythms and metabolism means that when you eat and exercise can be just as important as what you eat or how you exercise. Your body's ability to process food and utilize energy fluctuates throughout the day, meaning that the timing of your meals can affect everything from blood sugar levels to fat storage. Several studies have shown that eating more calories earlier in the day, when your metabolism is at its peak, can promote weight loss and improve metabolic health. This aligns with the concept of "front-loading" your calories—consuming a larger breakfast and lunch, and a smaller dinner. When you eat most of your calories during the day, your body is better able to burn energy, as insulin sensitivity is highest in the morning and decreases as the day progresses. This is why eating late at night, when your metabolism has slowed, can lead to fat storage and weight gain. Aligning your eating patterns with your circadian rhythm can improve digestion. Your digestive system follows its own daily cycle, with digestive enzymes and bile production peaking during the day and slowing down at night. This means your body is primed to handle and digest food more effectively during the daytime, while eating late at night can strain your digestive system, leading to discomfort and poor nutrient absorption. Just as meal timing matters, so does the timing of physical activity. Research suggests that exercising at certain times of the day can maximize your performance and metabolic benefits. While the "best" time to exercise can vary depending on individual preferences and schedules, late morning and early afternoon are often considered optimal times for physical performance. This is when your body temperature is higher, reaction times are faster, and muscle function is at its peak, all of which contribute to better endurance, strength, and flexibility. Morning exercise can also have its advantages, particularly when it comes to setting the tone for your day. Physical activity early in the morning can help regulate your circadian rhythm by signaling to your body that it's time to wake up and get moving. This can boost your energy levels, improve your mood, and promote better sleep at night. Additionally, some studies suggest that morning exercise can lead to better fat burning, as your body may be more inclined to use stored fat for energy after an overnight fast.

On the other hand, if you're someone who exercises in the evening, be mindful of how close to bedtime you're working out. While moderate exercise in the late afternoon can improve sleep quality, intense workouts too close to bedtime can interfere with your ability to fall asleep by raising your body temperature and stimulating your nervous system. For evening exercisers, it's important to cool down properly and allow at least a couple of hours for your body to wind down before hitting the pillow.

Strategies for Aligning with Natural Rhythms

Now that we understand how circadian rhythms influence sleep, metabolism, and physical performance, it's time to explore strategies to better align your daily habits with your natural rhythms. The goal is to create a routine that supports your body's biological clock, allowing it to function optimally and promote better health.

1.   Prioritize Consistent Sleep Patterns

The foundation of a healthy circadian rhythm starts with consistent sleep patterns. Aim to go to bed and wake up at the same time every day, even on weekends. This consistency helps regulate your body's internal clock, making it easier to fall asleep and wake up naturally. It also ensures that your body gets adequate time in each stage of the sleep cycle, supporting overall health.

2.   Embrace Natural Light Exposure

One of the most powerful ways to reset your circadian rhythm is by exposing yourself to natural light, particularly in the morning. Sunlight helps signal to your SCN that it's time to wake up, boosting cortisol production and suppressing melatonin. Aim to spend time outdoors in the early hours of the day or, if that's not possible, try to let in as much natural light as you can. Conversely, limit exposure to artificial light, especially blue light from screens, in the evening to encourage melatonin production and prepare your body for sleep.

3.   Time Your Meals Wisely

As mentioned earlier, the timing of your meals can have a significant impact on your metabolism. Try to align your eating schedule with your body's natural metabolic peaks by consuming larger meals earlier in the day. Avoid eating late at night, as this can disrupt your circadian rhythm and lead to metabolic dysfunction. If possible, aim to finish your last meal of the day at least two to three hours before bedtime to give your body enough time to digest food before sleep.

4.   Schedule Exercise According to Your Energy Levels

Exercise is another activity that can be timed according to your circadian rhythm. If you're a morning person, capitalize on that natural energy boost and fit in a workout early in the day. If you find you have more energy later on, aim for a mid-afternoon workout when your body temperature and muscle function are at their peak. Just be mindful of evening workouts, as they can sometimes interfere with sleep if done too close to bedtime.

5.   Incorporate Mindfulness Practices

Stress is a significant disruptor of circadian rhythms, as it elevates cortisol levels and interferes with sleep. Incorporating mindfulness practices like meditation, deep breathing, or yoga can help reduce stress and keep your circadian rhythm in balance. These activities also encourage relaxation, making it easier to transition into rest mode when it's time to sleep.

3.3 Managing Stress and Health

Stress is an inescapable part of life. While some stress is normal and even beneficial in certain situations, chronic or unmanaged stress can have serious consequences for your health—particularly for your metabolism. The connection between stress and metabolism is complex, influencing how your body processes food, stores fat, and regulates energy. But it's not just about how stress impacts your waistline; it also affects your mental well-being, cognitive function, and long-term physical health.

In this section, we will explore how stress affects your metabolism, practical techniques to manage stress effectively, and the role of mindfulness and meditation in fostering mental resilience and physical well-being.

The Connection Between Stress and Metabolism

When you experience stress, your body reacts by activating a system called the hypothalamic-pituitary-adrenal (HPA) axis. This system controls your stress response by releasing stress hormones such as cortisol and adrenaline. These hormones prepare your body for a "fight-or-flight" response, a mechanism that was crucial for our ancestors when facing immediate dangers like predators. Although the threats we face today may be different—deadlines at work, financial concerns, family responsibilities—our bodies still respond with the same biochemical reactions. In the short term, stress hormones can help you focus, increase your energy levels, and sharpen your reflexes. But when stress becomes chronic, these hormones remain elevated, creating imbalances in your body that can have harmful effects. One of the most well-known consequences of prolonged stress is its impact on metabolism. Cortisol, often referred to as the "stress hormone," plays a key role in how your body regulates fat, protein, and carbohydrate metabolism. Under acute stress, cortisol helps your body release glucose (sugar) into the bloodstream to provide immediate energy. However, when stress persists, cortisol remains elevated, which can disrupt your body's ability to process glucose effectively. Over time, this can lead to insulin resistance, a condition where your body's cells become less responsive to insulin, leading to higher blood sugar levels and, eventually, weight gain, especially around the abdominal area. Stress also affects your appetite. For some people, stress may suppress hunger temporarily, but for many, chronic stress triggers emotional eating or cravings for high-calorie, sugary, and fatty foods. This is because cortisol enhances the brain's reward centers, making these comfort foods more appealing. Combined with a sedentary lifestyle, these cravings can contribute to weight gain and other metabolic imbalances.

In addition to its effects on blood sugar and appetite, chronic stress can disrupt your sleep patterns. Sleep, as we've explored in earlier chapters, is essential for maintaining metabolic health. When you don't get enough sleep, or the quality of your sleep is poor, your body becomes less efficient at processing food and burning calories. Lack of sleep also leads to higher cortisol levels, creating a vicious cycle where stress begets poor sleep, and poor sleep begets more stress. The long-term effects of chronic stress on metabolism are not limited to weight gain. Research has shown that prolonged stress can increase the risk of developing metabolic syndrome—a cluster of conditions that include high blood pressure, high blood sugar, abnormal cholesterol levels, and excess body fat around the waist. Metabolic syndrome is a significant risk factor for heart disease, stroke, and type 2 diabetes, highlighting the importance of managing stress effectively to protect both your metabolic and cardiovascular health.

Stress Management Techniques

While it's impossible to eliminate stress entirely, there are numerous strategies you can use to manage it in healthy ways, helping to mitigate its negative effects on your metabolism and overall health. The goal of stress management isn't to avoid stress completely but to change how you respond to it, transforming it into a tool for growth and resilience. One of the most effective approaches to managing stress is by adopting regular physical activity. Exercise not only helps to burn calories and improve metabolic function, but it also acts as a natural stress reliever. Physical activity prompts the release of endorphins, often referred to as the brain's "feel-good" chemicals, which reduce the perception of pain and trigger positive feelings. Moreover, regular exercise lowers cortisol levels, helping to counteract the metabolic effects of chronic stress. It's important to find a form of exercise that you enjoy—whether it's jogging, swimming, yoga, or weight training—so that it becomes a sustainable habit.

Another key aspect of stress management is maintaining a healthy work-life balance. Many people experience chronic stress due to the pressures of work, often finding it difficult to set boundaries between their professional and personal lives. Taking time to recharge and disconnect from work is essential for reducing stress and protecting your health. Whether it's through hobbies, spending time with loved ones, or simply enjoying quiet moments of solitude, prioritizing relaxation can help restore balance and improve your mental and physical well-being.

Social support is another important factor in managing stress. Humans are inherently social creatures, and the connections we build with others can provide emotional strength during difficult times. Studies have shown that people with strong social networks tend to experience lower levels of stress and better overall health. Whether it's through friendships, family relationships, or community involvement, fostering meaningful connections can buffer the effects of stress and promote resilience. In addition to exercise, work-life balance, and social support, stress management can benefit from incorporating techniques that promote relaxation and mental clarity. Practices such as deep breathing, progressive muscle relaxation, and visualization exercises are simple yet effective ways to calm your mind and body in moments of acute stress. These techniques can be done almost anywhere and require no special equipment, making them accessible for anyone looking to reduce tension in a short amount of time. Time management is another practical approach to stress reduction. Many people feel overwhelmed by the sheer volume of tasks they need to complete, leading to heightened stress levels. Learning to prioritize tasks, break them into smaller, more manageable steps, and delegate when possible can significantly reduce feelings of overwhelm. Using tools such as planners, to-do lists, or apps that help track your progress can also enhance your productivity and free up time for relaxation.

Mindfulness and Meditation Practices

Mindfulness and meditation have gained widespread attention in recent years for their ability to reduce stress, improve mental health, and even enhance metabolic function. These practices involve paying attention to the present moment, without judgment, and can be powerful tools for managing stress and improving your overall sense of well-being.

Mindfulness, at its core, is about bringing awareness to your thoughts, emotions, and sensations in the present moment. By observing these experiences without trying to change or avoid them, mindfulness helps you develop a more balanced and accepting relationship with stress. Rather than reacting automatically to stressful situations, mindfulness encourages you to pause, reflect, and respond more thoughtfully. This can lead to better decision-making, improved emotional regulation, and a greater sense of calm.

One of the most popular mindfulness techniques is mindful breathing. In moments of stress, your breathing tends to become shallow and rapid, signaling to your body that you're in a state of distress. By practicing mindful breathing, you can activate the body's relaxation response, slowing your heart rate, lowering blood pressure, and reducing cortisol levels. A simple way to practice mindful breathing is to focus your attention on your breath as it enters and leaves your body, taking slow, deep breaths in through your nose and out through your mouth. Meditation is another practice closely related to mindfulness. While there are many different forms of meditation, most involve sitting quietly, focusing on your breath or a specific mantra, and allowing thoughts to come and go without attaching to them. Over time, regular meditation can help reduce stress, improve focus, and even lower cortisol levels, making it a valuable tool for managing the effects of chronic stress on your metabolism. Studies have shown that mindfulness and meditation not only reduce stress but also have direct effects on metabolism. For example, research suggests that practicing mindfulness can lower levels of cortisol, insulin resistance, and even inflammation—all of which are associated with metabolic health. By incorporating mindfulness into your daily routine, you can support your body's natural ability to regulate stress and maintain a healthy metabolism. Mindfulness and meditation practices can also improve your relationship with food, helping to reduce emotional eating and promote more mindful eating habits. When you eat mindfully, you pay attention to the sensory experience of eating—how the food looks, smells, tastes, and feels. This can help you tune into your body's hunger and fullness cues, making it easier to stop eating when you're satisfied, rather than overeating in response to stress or emotions. Stress is an unavoidable part of life, but how you manage it makes all the difference in its impact on your health. Understanding the connection between stress and metabolism can help you take proactive steps to protect your metabolic health and overall well-being. By incorporating regular exercise, fostering social connections, practicing mindfulness, and implementing relaxation techniques, you can reduce the harmful effects of chronic stress and support a healthier, more balanced lifestyle. Remember, stress is not the enemy—how you respond to it is what matters most.

3.4 The Importance of Active Recovery

In the pursuit of health and wellness, it is often easy to overlook the significance of recovery. While many focus on intense workouts and rigorous routines, the true path to improved fitness and metabolic health lies not just in hard work but also in how we allow our bodies to recuperate. Active recovery, a concept that promotes light activity after periods of exertion, plays a crucial role in overall well-being and is essential for optimizing both physical and mental health. Active recovery is distinct from complete rest; it involves engaging in low-intensity activities that keep the body moving without causing additional strain. This approach is particularly beneficial after high-intensity workouts or strenuous physical activities, where muscles are often left fatigued and in need of care. The act of recovery is not just about allowing your body to rest; it's about actively nurturing your body's systems to enhance performance, prevent injury, and support metabolic function.

Recovery Activities and Wellbeing

When we talk about recovery, it is important to understand its broader implications for our well-being. Engaging in recovery activities, whether they be physical or mental, can help enhance mood, reduce anxiety, and improve our overall outlook on life. This is especially relevant in today's fast-paced world, where stress is a common companion. Recovery is not merely a means to bounce back; it is an integral part of a holistic approach to health. Active recovery facilitates improved blood circulation, which is vital for delivering nutrients to muscles and removing waste products like lactic acid. This process not only aids in muscle repair but also reduces the likelihood of soreness, allowing you to return to your regular activities or workouts more quickly and efficiently. Moreover, engaging in light physical activities encourages the release of endorphins—our body's natural mood enhancers—providing both mental and physical benefits that can uplift spirits and promote a sense of well-being. Incorporating active recovery into your routine can also enhance flexibility and range of motion. Gentle activities, such as walking, yoga, or swimming, stretch and elongate muscles that may have become tight during high-intensity workouts. This is crucial for maintaining a healthy, functional body that is less prone to injuries. By nurturing flexibility, we not only improve our physical capabilities but also pave the way for a more enjoyable and sustainable exercise experience. The benefits of active recovery extend beyond the physical realm. It fosters a more mindful approach to our bodies and their needs. By tuning into how we feel post-exercise, we can better recognize signs of fatigue, overtraining, or potential injury. This awareness can lead to more informed decisions regarding our fitness routines and overall lifestyle, ensuring that we prioritize not just intensity but also the quality of our recovery.

Light Exercises and Stretching

Integrating light exercises into your active recovery regimen is one of the most effective strategies for promoting overall health. Activities such as walking or cycling at a leisurely pace can stimulate circulation and help keep your muscles engaged without the stress of high-intensity efforts. The beauty of light exercise lies in its simplicity; it can be easily woven into daily life, transforming what might otherwise be sedentary time into productive, health-promoting activity. Yoga and stretching are particularly powerful tools in the active recovery arsenal. Not only do they enhance flexibility and muscle relaxation, but they also encourage deep, mindful breathing, which can help to further reduce stress. Taking time to stretch after a workout or even on a rest day can alleviate tightness in muscles and joints, enhancing recovery and preparing your body for the next challenge. Stretching is not merely an act of physical rehabilitation; it is a practice that fosters awareness of our bodies. By focusing on different muscle groups, we learn to identify areas of tension or discomfort, which can inform our approach to future workouts. Additionally, incorporating regular stretching routines can create a soothing ritual that calms the mind and body, enhancing overall recovery. It is vital to listen to your body during active recovery. Everyone's needs will vary based on individual fitness levels, activity types, and overall health. Some may benefit from more vigorous forms of light exercise, while others may find solace in gentle yoga or leisurely strolls. The key is to respect your body's signals and engage in activities that feel rejuvenating rather than taxing.

Incorporating Rest into Your Routine

Creating a routine that prioritizes active recovery is crucial for long-term health and fitness success. This involves not just scheduling workouts but also recognizing the importance of rest as part of that schedule. Incorporating dedicated recovery days or periods into your week can significantly enhance your physical and mental performance. One of the most effective ways to integrate active recovery into your routine is by planning specific days or times where the focus shifts from intensity to restorative practices. This could mean designating certain days for light activities, or it could involve incorporating short recovery sessions within your existing workout regimen. For instance, you might include a 10- to 15-minute session of stretching or yoga following your main workout. This not only aids recovery but can also become an enjoyable transition that allows you to wind down after a rigorous session. Consider the environmental factors that contribute to your recovery. Creating a space conducive to relaxation—whether at home or in a gym—can enhance your experience. This could involve playing calming music, utilizing soft lighting, or simply being in a peaceful outdoor setting. When we create an environment that promotes relaxation and recuperation, we are more likely to engage in these practices regularly. In addition to structured recovery periods, you might also incorporate spontaneous moments of rest throughout your day. This could involve taking a few minutes to stretch during breaks at work, going for a gentle walk after lunch, or practicing mindful breathing exercises before bed. These small actions can accumulate over time, creating a holistic approach to recovery that seamlessly integrates into your lifestyle. Recognizing the importance of active recovery empowers you to take charge of your health. It fosters a deeper connection to your body, allowing you to navigate the challenges of exercise with awareness and intention. By balancing effort with recovery, you cultivate a sustainable approach to fitness that can support your metabolic health and overall well-being for years to come. Active recovery is a vital component of any fitness regimen, serving as a bridge between the demands of physical exertion and the need for rest. By engaging in light exercises and stretching, you enhance your body's natural ability to recover while simultaneously nurturing your mental well-being. Incorporating rest into your routine not only supports your physical health but also cultivates a mindset that prioritizes self-care, balance, and long-term sustainability in your fitness journey.

3.5 Creating a Healthy Sleep Environment

Creating a healthy sleep environment is foundational to achieving restful and restorative sleep, which in turn plays a pivotal role in overall health and well-being. The space where we sleep has a profound impact on the quality of our rest, and by thoughtfully designing this environment, we can enhance our sleep experience and, subsequently, our waking lives.

Factors Affecting Sleep

Many factors contribute to the quality of our sleep, ranging from external elements like light and noise to internal ones such as stress and anxiety. Understanding these influences can empower us to make informed adjustments that promote better sleep. One of the most significant external factors is light exposure. Our bodies are wired to respond to natural light cycles, and exposure to bright lights, particularly blue light emitted by screens, can disrupt the production of melatonin, the hormone responsible for regulating sleep. This disruption can lead to difficulties in falling asleep, reduced sleep duration, and poorer sleep quality. Therefore, creating a dimly lit environment in the hour leading up to bedtime can signal to our bodies that it's time to wind down. Noise is another critical factor that can interfere with our sleep. While some people may find white noise soothing, others may be more sensitive to disturbances, which can lead to fragmented sleep and daytime fatigue. External sounds like traffic, neighbors, or even household activities can invade our sleep space, making it essential to create an environment that minimizes these disruptions. Soundproofing elements, such as heavy curtains or even earplugs, can help create a more tranquil sleeping atmosphere. Temperature also plays a crucial role in sleep quality. Studies suggest that cooler sleeping environments—generally between 60 and 67 degrees Fahrenheit—are optimal for achieving deeper sleep. When the body temperature drops slightly during sleep, it encourages a more restorative state. Therefore, adjusting the thermostat, using breathable bedding, and choosing appropriate sleepwear can make a significant difference in how well we rest. The psychological aspects of our sleep environment should not be overlooked. Our bedroom should be a sanctuary, a place where we feel safe, relaxed, and comfortable. Clutter and chaos can create feelings of anxiety and restlessness, making it more challenging to drift off. By maintaining a tidy and organized space, we can foster a more peaceful atmosphere conducive to sleep.

How to Optimize Your Bedroom

Optimizing your bedroom for sleep involves creating an inviting and calming space. Start with your bed, which is the centerpiece of your sleeping environment. Investing in a quality mattress and pillows that provide the right level of support can make a world of difference. Comfort is paramount; if you find yourself tossing and turning, it may be time to evaluate your bedding choices. Next, consider the decor and color scheme of your bedroom. Soft, neutral colors can evoke a sense of calm, while bright, bold colors may stimulate the mind and make it harder to relax. Incorporating elements of nature—such as plants or natural wood—can also promote tranquility and a connection to the outdoors, which has been shown to enhance relaxation and reduce stress. Lighting is another vital component of a sleep-friendly environment. Consider using blackout curtains to prevent outside light from seeping in. Additionally, utilizing dimmable lights or bedside lamps with warm bulbs can help create a soft, cozy atmosphere in the evenings. The goal is to cultivate a space that transitions seamlessly from the busyness of daytime to the calm of nighttime. Air quality is equally important. Ensure your bedroom is well-ventilated, as fresh air promotes better sleep. You might consider using an air purifier to reduce allergens and pollutants that can disrupt your breathing during the night. Maintaining a clean sleeping space, free from dust and allergens, is essential for fostering a healthy sleep environment.

Creating a bedtime routine can further enhance your sleep environment. Engage in calming activities before bed, such as reading, meditating, or taking a warm bath. These practices signal to your body that it is time to wind down, making it easier to transition into sleep. Setting a consistent sleep schedule, where you go to bed and wake up at the same time each day, reinforces your body's natural circadian rhythms, promoting deeper and more restorative sleep.

Tips for Good Sleep Hygiene

Good sleep hygiene is not just about creating the right environment; it also involves cultivating habits that promote restful sleep. Start by limiting exposure to screens in the hour before bed. The blue light emitted by smartphones, tablets, and computers can interfere with your body's natural production of melatonin. Consider establishing a digital curfew, allowing your mind to detach from technology and unwind before sleep. Nutrition also plays a significant role in sleep hygiene. Avoid large meals and heavy, rich foods close to bedtime, as they can lead to discomfort and disrupt sleep. Instead, opt for lighter snacks if you're hungry, such as a small serving of yogurt or a piece of fruit. Be mindful of caffeine and alcohol consumption. Caffeine can linger in your system for hours, making it harder to fall asleep, while alcohol may initially induce drowsiness but can disrupt sleep cycles later in the night. Regular physical activity contributes positively to sleep quality, but timing is key. Engaging in vigorous exercise too close to bedtime can have a stimulating effect, making it harder to wind down. Aim to complete workouts earlier in the day or at least a few hours before bed. Conversely, gentle exercises, such as yoga or stretching, can promote relaxation and prepare your body for sleep. Stress and anxiety can significantly impact sleep quality, making it essential to incorporate relaxation techniques into your bedtime routine. Deep breathing exercises, progressive muscle relaxation, or mindfulness meditation can help calm the mind and body, allowing you to drift off more peacefully. Creating a healthy sleep environment involves a multifaceted approach that encompasses the physical space of your bedroom as well as your daily habits and routines. By paying attention to factors such as light, noise, temperature, and cleanliness, you can design a sanctuary that supports restful sleep. Coupled with good sleep hygiene practices, such as limiting screen time, mindful nutrition, and managing stress, you can significantly enhance the quality of your sleep. As you prioritize your sleep environment, you are investing in your overall health and well-being, leading to greater vitality and resilience in your daily life.

program that addresses cardiovascular health, muscle strength, and joint mobility. This holistic approach can be particularly beneficial for older adults seeking to maintain their independence and functional capacity as they age.

Cardiovascular vs. Strength Training

The debate between cardiovascular exercise and strength training is a longstanding one, with proponents on both sides advocating for their respective benefits. While these two forms of exercise may seem distinct, they complement one another, forming the foundation of a balanced fitness routine. Cardiovascular training is often celebrated for its ability to improve heart health and endurance. The rhythmic nature of activities like jogging or swimming can elevate your heart rate, making your heart work more efficiently over time. As you engage in consistent cardiovascular exercise, you may notice improvements in your stamina. Consider a person training for a half-marathon. They start with short runs and gradually increase their distance, learning to pace themselves and build endurance. This journey not only prepares their body for the event but also instills a sense of accomplishment as they witness their progress. The endorphin release during these sessions often leads to a greater sense of well-being, reducing feelings of anxiety and depression. Conversely, strength training focuses on building muscle mass and enhancing metabolic function. As muscle tissue grows, the body becomes more efficient at burning calories, even when at rest. Imagine a middle-aged woman who begins lifting weights at her local gym. Initially, she struggles to complete her sets, but with perseverance, she develops noticeable muscle tone and strength. Her metabolism increases, making it easier to manage her weight while enjoying her favorite foods without guilt. Additionally, strength training promotes bone density, a crucial aspect of health as we age, protecting against osteoporosis and fractures.

While both forms of exercise offer unique advantages, their combined effects can lead to extraordinary results. For instance, an individual who participates in both cardiovascular and strength training will likely experience improved overall fitness. The aerobic component enhances endurance, while strength training builds the muscular foundation necessary for functional movements in daily life. A person who engages in both might find themselves able to climb a flight of stairs without becoming winded, all while carrying groceries—a perfect example of how the two forms of exercise work together.

In essence, rather than pitting these exercises against each other, it's more beneficial to recognize their complementary nature. Individuals aiming for weight loss or improved fitness should consider incorporating both into their routine. This balanced approach not only maximizes benefits but also reduces the risk of overuse injuries that can arise from focusing too heavily on one type of exercise.

The Importance of Daily Movement

As we navigate our increasingly sedentary lives, the significance of daily movement cannot be overstated. It's easy to become ensnared in routines that involve prolonged periods of sitting—whether at a desk job, during commutes, or while binge-watching our favorite shows. Incorporating movement throughout the day is crucial for maintaining a healthy metabolism and overall well-being. Daily movement can take many forms. It doesn't have to involve structured workouts; instead, it can be integrated seamlessly into everyday activities. For instance, consider a typical office worker who decides to take short breaks every hour to stretch or walk around the office. These simple adjustments lead to increased circulation and energy levels. When this worker returns to their desk, they often find themselves more focused and productive, counteracting the sluggishness that comes from sitting for too long.

Think of how daily movement can also enhance social interactions. A group of friends who make it a habit to walk during their lunch breaks not only benefits from the physical activity but also deepens their relationships. Conversations flow more freely as they stroll through a nearby park, enjoying the fresh air and sunshine. This practice promotes not only physical fitness but also emotional well-being, showcasing how movement can enrich our lives in more ways than one.

The cumulative effect of small bursts of activity throughout the day can yield significant health benefits. Imagine a person who decides to park further away from the entrance of their workplace, consciously opting to take the stairs instead of the elevator. These small decisions may seem inconsequential at first, but over weeks and months, they contribute to increased calorie expenditure and improved cardiovascular health. When these choices become habitual, they foster a lifestyle centered around movement, creating a positive feedback loop that encourages even more activity. For those who may find it challenging to engage in longer workouts, focusing on daily movement can be a game-changer. A busy parent might not have time for an hour at the gym, but they can incorporate movement by playing actively with their children. Whether it's chasing after kids in the backyard or taking family walks in the evening, these moments of play foster connection while promoting health. Embracing daily movement is about adopting a mindset that values activity as a crucial component of life. By consciously integrating movement into our routines, we not only combat the negative effects of a sedentary lifestyle but also cultivate a greater appreciation for the physical capabilities of our bodies. Every step taken, every stretch performed, and every playful moment shared adds up to create a vibrant and fulfilling life.

Chapter 4: Physical Activity and Metabolism

4.1 Benefits of Regular Exercise

Types of Exercises and Their Effects

Physical activity comes in many forms, and understanding the effects of different types of exercises on the body and metabolism is key to optimizing your health. Broadly speaking, exercise can be divided into aerobic (cardiovascular) and anaerobic (strength training) categories, with each offering unique benefits to your metabolic health and overall fitness.

Aerobic exercise, also known as cardiovascular or endurance exercise, includes activities such as walking, running, cycling, swimming, and dancing. This type of exercise primarily uses oxygen to meet the energy demands of prolonged, moderate activity. Aerobic exercise improves cardiovascular and pulmonary health by enhancing the capacity of your heart and lungs to deliver oxygen to your muscles. As a result, it increases endurance and helps the body efficiently burn fat and carbohydrates for energy.

The impact of aerobic exercise on metabolism is particularly significant. It boosts your metabolic rate both during and after the activity, resulting in what's called the "afterburn effect." This means your body continues to burn calories at an elevated rate after you've completed your workout. Aerobic exercises are also essential for improving insulin sensitivity, which helps regulate blood sugar levels and reduce the risk of metabolic diseases such as type 2 diabetes.

On the other hand, **anaerobic exercise** involves short bursts of high-intensity activity, such as weightlifting, sprinting, and resistance training. These exercises do not rely primarily on oxygen for energy; instead, they use energy stored in your muscles. Strength training, a form of anaerobic exercise, is particularly beneficial for building muscle mass. Since muscle tissue is more metabolically active than fat tissue, having more muscle increases your resting metabolic rate (RMR). This means you'll burn more calories even when you're not exercising.

In addition to increasing metabolic rate, anaerobic exercises help improve bone density, muscle strength, and joint flexibility. They also contribute to better metabolic flexibility—the ability of your body to switch between burning fat and carbohydrates as needed for energy. This flexibility is important for maintaining energy levels and supporting long-term metabolic health.

Both types of exercises play a crucial role in enhancing metabolic health. By incorporating a mix of aerobic and anaerobic activities into your fitness routine, you can target different aspects of metabolism and create a balanced, sustainable approach to improving your overall health.

Cardiovascular vs. Strength Training

The distinction between cardiovascular (aerobic) and strength (anaerobic) training is often discussed in terms of their specific benefits to the body and metabolism. While they may appear to serve different purposes, both are equally important for maintaining a healthy, well-functioning metabolism.

Cardiovascular exercise focuses on improving your heart and lung capacity. Activities like running, cycling, and swimming increase your heart rate, which in turn strengthens your cardiovascular system and enhances your body's ability to deliver oxygen to working muscles. This improvement in oxygen delivery is vital for efficient energy production at the cellular level. Over time, consistent cardiovascular exercise can lead to improved endurance, better circulation, and a lower resting heart rate—indicators of a strong and healthy cardiovascular system.

For metabolic health, cardio is especially effective at burning fat. As you engage in prolonged aerobic exercise, your body shifts to using fat as its primary source of energy, which helps reduce overall body fat percentage. This is particularly important for individuals looking to manage their weight or improve their body composition. Additionally, cardiovascular exercise helps regulate cholesterol levels and reduces the risk of heart disease, which is often linked to poor metabolic health.

In contrast, **strength training** targets the muscles, bones, and joints. Lifting weights or using resistance bands challenges your muscles to grow stronger, increasing muscle mass and bone density. Since muscle tissue burns more calories than fat, having more muscle significantly boosts your basal metabolic rate (BMR), meaning you'll burn more calories even at rest.

Strength training also improves insulin sensitivity and glucose metabolism, which helps stabilize blood sugar levels. This is particularly important for preventing or managing conditions like diabetes. Furthermore, resistance training enhances metabolic flexibility, allowing your body to efficiently switch between energy sources depending on your activity level and diet.

While cardiovascular exercise may burn more calories during the workout, strength training offers longer-lasting metabolic benefits due to its impact on muscle mass. For optimal health, it's important to strike a balance between both forms of exercise, ensuring your cardiovascular system stays strong while also maintaining and building muscle.

The Importance of Daily Movement

Beyond structured exercise, the importance of daily movement cannot be overstated. In today's increasingly sedentary lifestyle, where many people spend hours sitting at desks or in front of screens, incorporating regular physical movement throughout the day is critical for maintaining metabolic health.

Sitting for prolonged periods has been linked to a number of metabolic and cardiovascular issues, including weight gain, poor circulation, and increased risk of chronic diseases. This phenomenon is often referred to as "sitting disease," and it underscores the necessity of breaking up long periods of inactivity with movement.

Incorporating movement into daily life can be as simple as taking regular walking breaks, standing while working, or doing light stretching exercises throughout the day. These small, consistent efforts help to keep the body's energy systems engaged and prevent the negative metabolic effects of prolonged inactivity. Moving regularly throughout the day also helps maintain insulin sensitivity, keeping blood sugar levels stable, and encourages better circulation, which supports overall metabolic function.

Even activities such as taking the stairs instead of the elevator, parking further away from your destination, or doing household chores like gardening or cleaning can significantly contribute to your daily physical activity levels. These non-exercise physical activities, known as **NEAT** (non-exercise activity thermogenesis), play a vital role in maintaining metabolic health and preventing the gradual weight gain that can occur from a sedentary lifestyle.

Daily movement also supports **mental health**, reducing stress and promoting the release of endorphins, which help regulate mood and enhance feelings of well-being. Stress, if left unmanaged, can negatively impact metabolism by increasing levels of cortisol, a hormone associated with fat storage and poor metabolic function.

To promote daily movement, it's helpful to create a routine that includes both structured exercise and informal physical activities. For example, you might begin your day with a 30-minute walk or workout, followed by intermittent stretching or standing breaks during the workday. In the evening, engaging in light physical activities, such as playing with children, taking a walk after dinner, or doing yoga, can keep your body active and engaged.

For individuals with busy schedules, finding time to move can be challenging, but prioritizing even small moments of physical activity can have profound long-term health benefits. The key is to view movement not as an isolated task but as an integral part of your daily routine that supports both physical and metabolic well-being.

Remember, regular exercise plays an essential role in supporting metabolic health, and understanding the different types of exercises—cardiovascular and strength training—can help you develop a well-rounded fitness routine. Cardiovascular exercise improves endurance and fat-burning capacity, while strength training builds muscle and boosts long-term metabolic rate. Incorporating daily movement beyond structured workouts is equally important, as it helps combat the negative effects of a sedentary lifestyle and supports overall metabolic function. By making physical activity a priority, you can enjoy lasting benefits, including better energy levels, improved mood, and reduced risk of chronic diseases.

4.2 Building an Effective Exercise Routine

Designing an effective exercise routine is crucial for achieving lasting fitness and maintaining metabolic health. However, building a plan that is sustainable, enjoyable, and tailored to your individual needs can often be challenging. Whether you are just beginning your fitness journey or you're experienced but looking to refine your approach, planning a structured workout program involves more than simply choosing exercises. It requires setting realistic goals, maintaining motivation, and adapting your plan as needed based on age, fitness level, and personal circumstances.

How to Plan a Workout Program

The first step in creating an effective workout program is understanding your individual goals. Your objectives may vary—whether you aim to lose weight, build muscle, improve cardiovascular health, or enhance overall well-being. Regardless of your goals, it's important to begin with a clear vision of what you want to achieve and then design a plan that incorporates exercises and routines that align with those outcomes.

When planning your routine, consider the principle of **balance**. An effective workout program should include a mix of cardiovascular exercises, strength training, and flexibility work to ensure that you are targeting all the key components of physical fitness. Cardiovascular exercises, like running, cycling, or swimming, are essential for improving heart health and increasing your body's ability to burn fat. Strength training, such as lifting weights or bodyweight exercises, builds muscle mass and enhances metabolic rate. Meanwhile, flexibility work, which includes activities like yoga or stretching, helps prevent injury and maintains mobility, especially as you age.

It's also important to think about the **frequency** of your workouts. While there's no one-size-fits-all approach, most experts recommend exercising at least 3-5 times per week. The frequency should be balanced with intensity and duration, as overtraining can lead to burnout, injury, or diminished results. A well-rounded routine may involve alternating between more intense days, such as strength training or high-intensity interval training (HIIT), and lighter days focused on recovery or flexibility exercises.

Another critical element in planning your program is **progression**. Your body adapts to the stresses placed upon it, so it's essential to gradually increase the intensity, duration, or complexity of your workouts over time. This could mean lifting heavier weights, running longer distances, or introducing more challenging exercises as your strength and endurance improve. Progression is the key to continuous improvement, as it prevents plateaus and ensures that your body is constantly being challenged in new ways.

A successful exercise routine also needs to account for **rest and recovery**. While it might seem counterintuitive, rest days are just as important as workout days. Your muscles need time to repair and grow stronger after being stressed by physical activity. Without sufficient recovery, you risk overtraining, which can lead to injury, fatigue, and a drop in performance. Incorporating active recovery days—where you engage in low-intensity activities like walking, light yoga, or stretching—can help maintain consistency without overwhelming your body.

It's essential to **individualize** your workout program. What works for one person might not work for another, and this is where self-awareness becomes critical. Factors such as your current fitness level, any pre-existing health conditions, and your lifestyle should all influence your plan. Customizing your routine allows you to create a program that fits seamlessly into your daily life and increases the likelihood of long-term success.

Setting Goals and Staying Motivated

Setting realistic and measurable goals is perhaps one of the most important aspects of building an effective exercise routine. Goals give you something to aim for, helping to keep you focused and motivated along your fitness journey. However, the key is to set goals that are **SMART**—specific, measurable, achievable, relevant, and time-bound. For instance, instead of saying, "I want to get fit," you could set a specific goal like, "I want to run a 5K in under 30 minutes within the next three months." This type of goal provides a clear target and a deadline, making it easier to stay on track and measure your progress.

Short-term goals play a significant role in maintaining motivation. While your ultimate goal might be to lose 20 pounds or improve your marathon time, focusing on smaller, more immediate objectives—like completing three workouts this week or increasing your squat weight by 10 pounds—can help sustain your motivation along the way. These small victories not only provide a sense of accomplishment but also help reinforce positive behaviors.

In addition to setting achievable goals, it's important to **celebrate progress**. Recognizing your achievements, no matter how small, can be incredibly motivating. Progress is not always linear, and fitness journeys are often filled with ups and downs. Learning to appreciate the journey and celebrate milestones, such as lifting a heavier weight or completing a longer run, can help maintain momentum even when results aren't immediately visible.

Another way to stay motivated is by varying your routine. **Monotony** is one of the biggest enemies of motivation in fitness. Doing the same workout day in and day out can lead to boredom, making it easier to skip sessions or lose interest. By incorporating variety into your program—whether through new exercises, different workout formats, or even changing the environment in which you exercise—you can keep things fresh and exciting. For example, instead of always running on a treadmill, try running outside, or switch between weight training and bodyweight exercises to keep your muscles guessing.

It's also helpful to have a **support system**. Whether it's a workout buddy, a personal trainer, or an online fitness community, having people to share your progress with and keep you accountable can be a powerful motivator. Exercising with others can provide both encouragement and healthy competition, which helps you push yourself to new levels. If you're working out solo, logging your progress on fitness apps or sharing it on social media can offer the same sense of accountability and motivation.

Finally, the **psychological aspect** of motivation should not be overlooked. Many people struggle with self-discipline, especially when they don't see immediate results. It's important to remember that fitness is a long-term commitment and that consistency is key. To combat the tendency to quit, try adopting a growth mindset. Recognize that setbacks are part of the process and that persistence, rather than perfection, will ultimately lead to success.

Adaptations for Different Ages and Fitness Levels

An effective workout routine should be adaptable for individuals of different ages and fitness levels. As we age, our bodies undergo natural changes, such as decreased muscle mass, reduced bone density, and a slower metabolism. However, these changes do not mean that fitness becomes less important—in fact, it becomes even more crucial to maintain a regular exercise routine that supports longevity and overall health.

For **younger adults** and those at a higher fitness level, a workout program may include higher-intensity exercises, such as HIIT, heavy weightlifting, or endurance sports like long-distance running. These individuals can handle more intense workouts and shorter recovery times, allowing for more frequent and vigorous exercise. The focus here is often on building strength, endurance, and cardiovascular fitness while maximizing metabolic rate.

For **middle-aged adults**, workouts may need to shift slightly to account for changes in muscle mass and joint flexibility. Strength training remains critical, but there may be a greater emphasis on flexibility and mobility exercises to ensure joint health and prevent injury. Cardiovascular exercise remains important, but individuals in this age group may benefit from moderate-intensity workouts that are gentler on the joints, such as cycling or swimming.

For **older adults**, exercise routines should focus on maintaining functional fitness—activities that improve strength, balance, and mobility, which are essential for daily tasks. Strength training can still be part of the routine, but it may involve lighter weights and more repetitions to prevent injury. Low-impact cardiovascular exercises like walking, swimming, or cycling are ideal for maintaining heart health without placing undue stress on the body. Flexibility exercises, such as yoga or Pilates, can help preserve mobility and prevent falls, a common concern in older populations.

Regardless of age, it's essential to listen to your body and adjust your routine accordingly. Exercise is not a one-size-fits-all solution, and what works for someone else may not be suitable for you. The key is to find a routine that challenges you while also being safe, enjoyable, and sustainable over the long term.

Building an effective exercise routine requires careful planning, goal setting, and the flexibility to adapt as you progress. By balancing various types of exercise, setting realistic goals, staying motivated, and tailoring your routine to your age and fitness level, you can create a program that supports both immediate and long-term health benefits. Remember, fitness is a journey, not a destination, and the most important factor in success is consistency. Keep moving, stay positive, and enjoy the process of becoming a healthier, stronger version of yourself.

4.3 Functional Training for Daily Life

Functional training has become an increasingly popular method for building strength, improving mobility, and enhancing the quality of daily life. Unlike traditional bodybuilding exercises that target specific muscles in isolation, functional training focuses on exercises that mimic the movements we use in everyday activities. The goal is to improve your body's ability to perform tasks such as lifting, bending, squatting, and reaching—movements that are essential for everything from household chores to recreational activities. This type of training not only strengthens your muscles but also enhances coordination, balance, and flexibility, ensuring that you can move efficiently and without injury throughout the day.

Practical Resistance Exercises

One of the key components of functional training is the use of **resistance exercises**. These exercises challenge your muscles to work against an external force, which can be anything from your body weight to resistance bands or free weights. The primary difference between functional resistance exercises and more traditional strength training is that the former engages multiple muscle groups at once, encouraging your body to work as a unit rather than in isolated parts.

Squats are a perfect example of a practical resistance exercise. In daily life, squatting is essential for sitting down, standing up, or picking objects off the ground. Performing squats as part of your training routine strengthens your legs, hips, and core, all of which are crucial for stability and balance. To perform a proper squat, stand with your feet shoulder-width apart, engage your core, and lower yourself as if sitting back into a chair. Keep your chest up and knees aligned with your toes. Once you reach a comfortable depth, press through your heels to stand back up. This movement mirrors everyday activities and helps build functional strength.

Another practical exercise is the **lunge**, which mimics the movement of walking or climbing stairs. Lunges strengthen the legs and improve balance, making it easier to navigate uneven surfaces or move from one position to another. To perform a lunge, step forward with one foot and lower your body until both knees are bent at 90 degrees. Push back up through your front foot to return to the starting position, and then repeat with the other leg. Lunges can be done with or without added resistance, such as holding dumbbells or using a resistance band.

The **deadlift** is another functional resistance exercise that teaches proper lifting mechanics, reducing the risk of injury when lifting heavy objects in daily life. In a deadlift, you bend at your hips while keeping your back straight, then lift a weight from the floor by engaging your legs, hips, and core. This movement strengthens the posterior chain—the muscles along the back of your body—including the hamstrings, glutes, and lower back. These muscles are essential for maintaining good posture and preventing lower back pain, especially during activities that involve lifting or bending.

Lastly, **push-ups** are a classic example of a bodyweight resistance exercise that mimics pushing movements used in daily activities, such as opening doors or moving heavy objects. Push-ups engage the chest, shoulders, triceps, and core, making them a versatile and functional exercise that strengthens the upper body while improving core stability.

Incorporating these practical resistance exercises into your routine helps build strength in a way that directly benefits your daily life. The focus is not on how much weight you can lift but on how efficiently and safely your body moves through space, reducing the risk of injury and improving overall performance.

Incorporating Movement into Your Routine

One of the advantages of functional training is that it can easily be integrated into your daily routine. Unlike gym-based workouts that require dedicated time and equipment, functional exercises often mimic the movements you already perform, making them more adaptable to your lifestyle. By simply being mindful of your movement throughout the day, you can turn everyday activities into opportunities to improve your fitness.

For example, instead of bending over to pick up an object, try using a proper **squat or lunge**. Not only does this strengthen your legs and core, but it also helps prevent back strain from poor lifting techniques. Similarly, when carrying groceries or other heavy items, engage your core and use a **farmer's carry** technique—holding the weights close to your body with a neutral spine. This movement is highly functional as it mirrors tasks like carrying suitcases, grocery bags, or even children.

When sitting for long periods, incorporate **mini-breaks** where you stand up, stretch, or perform a few bodyweight squats or lunges. This encourages blood flow, reduces stiffness, and engages muscles that might otherwise be inactive during prolonged sitting. Even simple tasks like standing on one leg while brushing your teeth can help improve balance and stability.

Another way to integrate functional movement is through **active transportation**. Instead of driving everywhere, walk or bike to nearby destinations. Walking is a low-impact, functional movement that improves cardiovascular health and strengthens the lower body. If you must drive, park farther away from your destination to increase the amount of walking you do throughout the day.

For those who work in an office or have sedentary jobs, standing desks can be a great way to incorporate movement into your workday. Alternating between sitting and standing helps reduce the negative effects of prolonged sitting, such as decreased metabolism and poor posture. You can also use your breaks to do quick **mobility exercises**, like shoulder rolls or hip stretches, which help maintain flexibility and prevent stiffness.

Home Exercise Examples

One of the greatest benefits of functional training is that it can be done anywhere, including the comfort of your own home. You don't need expensive gym equipment to build a functional workout routine—many effective exercises can be performed using just your body weight or a few simple tools like resistance bands or light dumbbells.

A simple yet effective exercise for home is the **plank**. Planks engage your entire core, helping to build the strength and stability needed for virtually every movement in daily life, from lifting objects to maintaining proper posture. To perform a plank, start in a push-up position, but instead of lowering yourself to the floor, hold your body in a straight line from head to heels, with your elbows under your shoulders. Engage your core and hold the position for as long as possible, focusing on keeping your hips level and avoiding sagging in the lower back. The plank strengthens the core, back, and shoulders, making it an essential part of any functional routine.

Another excellent home exercise is the **step-up**. If you have stairs or a sturdy step, this exercise mimics the action of climbing, which is a highly functional movement. Step-ups strengthen the legs and improve balance while also challenging the core for stability. To perform a step-up, place one foot on the step, push through your heel, and lift your body up until your leg is fully extended. Lower back down with control and repeat on the other side. For added resistance, you can hold dumbbells or a kettlebell.

A great full-body functional exercise is the **bear crawl**. This exercise engages your entire body, focusing on core stability, shoulder strength, and coordination. To perform a bear crawl, start on all fours with your hands directly under your shoulders and knees under your hips. Lift your knees off the floor so only your hands and feet are in contact with the ground. Slowly crawl forward, moving your opposite hand and foot together. This movement replicates the natural crawling motion and strengthens the muscles needed for stability and coordination in everyday activities.

If you have a resistance band, **banded rows** are a great home exercise for strengthening the upper back and improving posture. To perform a banded row, loop the band around a sturdy object and hold the ends in each hand. Step back to create tension in the band, then pull the handles towards your torso, squeezing your shoulder blades together as you do so. This exercise mimics pulling movements used in daily life, such as opening doors or lifting objects.

Functional training at home is not only convenient but also highly effective for improving strength, mobility, and coordination. By focusing on movements that replicate daily activities, you can create a workout routine that prepares your body for the demands of everyday life while enhancing your overall health and fitness.

Functional training offers a practical and efficient approach to fitness, emphasizing movements that replicate the demands of daily life. By incorporating practical resistance exercises, finding ways to integrate movement into your routine, and utilizing home exercises, you can build strength, improve mobility, and enhance your overall quality of life. Whether you're performing squats to strengthen your legs or using bodyweight exercises like planks and bear crawls to build core stability, functional training provides a versatile and effective solution for maintaining long-term health and fitness.

4.4 The Impact of Posture on Health

Posture plays a critical role in maintaining overall health and well-being. While it's often overlooked, poor posture can lead to a wide range of physical issues, including chronic pain, decreased mobility, and even metabolic inefficiencies. Conversely, good posture supports proper alignment of the spine and muscles, improves breathing, and allows the body to function more efficiently in everyday tasks. Understanding the impact of posture on health and implementing strategies to improve it can dramatically enhance your quality of life.

Recognizing Poor Posture

The first step to improving posture is being able to recognize the signs of poor alignment. Poor posture often develops gradually over time due to habits like sitting for prolonged periods, using smartphones or computers with a hunched back, or lifting objects with improper mechanics. It can lead to imbalances in the muscles, with some becoming overly tight and others weakening. These imbalances can cause discomfort, restricted movement, and, if left unaddressed, chronic pain.

One of the most common signs of poor posture is **forward head posture**, sometimes referred to as "tech neck." This occurs when the head juts forward in relation to the shoulders, often as a result of prolonged time spent looking at screens. This misalignment places strain on the neck and upper back, leading to tension headaches, neck pain, and discomfort in the shoulders. Another prevalent issue is **rounded shoulders**, where the upper back slumps forward, causing the chest to collapse inward. This posture restricts lung capacity and can lead to shallow breathing, as well as tension in the upper back and neck.

Lower body posture can also suffer from daily habits, particularly in seated positions. **Anterior pelvic tilt**, where the pelvis tilts forward and creates an excessive curve in the lower back, is another common issue. This is often seen in people who spend long hours sitting, causing tight hip flexors and a weakened core. It can lead to lower back pain and strain on the lumbar spine.

When poor posture becomes habitual, the body compensates by relying on the wrong muscles to perform movements, increasing the risk of injury. These compensations can disrupt the body's natural alignment, affecting everything from joint function to the efficiency of your metabolism. For example, poor posture can restrict breathing, limiting oxygen intake and reducing the effectiveness of physical activity.

Recognizing poor posture involves being mindful of how you sit, stand, and move throughout the day. Take note of whether your head is aligned over your shoulders, whether your shoulders are rolled forward, and if you frequently experience tension or discomfort in your neck, back, or hips. Becoming aware of these patterns is the first step toward correcting them.

Exercises to Improve Posture

Improving posture involves strengthening the muscles that support proper alignment while stretching those that may have become tight or shortened due to poor habits. Incorporating specific exercises into your routine can help correct imbalances, restore natural alignment, and prevent further complications.

One of the most effective exercises for improving posture is the **plank**, which strengthens the core muscles responsible for maintaining a neutral spine. To perform a plank, place your forearms on the ground with your elbows directly under your shoulders and your body in a straight line from head to heels. Engage your core and hold this position, focusing on keeping your hips level and avoiding sagging in the lower back. A strong core is essential for maintaining good posture, as it supports the spine and prevents excessive curvature in the lower back.

Wall angels are another excellent exercise for improving upper body posture. To perform this movement, stand with your back against a wall, keeping your feet about six inches away from the base of the wall. Press your lower back, upper back, and head against the wall, and bring your arms up to a 90-degree angle, with your elbows and hands touching the wall. Slowly raise and lower your arms, keeping your entire body in contact with the wall. This exercise helps correct rounded shoulders by engaging the muscles of the upper back and shoulders, promoting better alignment.

The **cat-cow stretch**, a yoga-inspired movement, is highly effective for mobilizing the spine and relieving tension in the lower back. Begin on all fours, with your hands directly under your shoulders and your knees under your hips. As you inhale, arch your back, lifting your chest and tailbone toward the ceiling (cow pose). On the exhale, round your back, tucking your chin to your chest and drawing your belly button toward your spine (cat pose). This dynamic movement encourages spinal flexibility and can help counteract the stiffness and discomfort associated with poor posture, particularly in the lower back.

Another key exercise is the **bridge**, which strengthens the glutes and hamstrings while stretching the hip flexors. To perform the bridge, lie on your back with your knees bent and feet flat on the floor. Engage your core and press through your heels to lift your hips off the ground, forming a straight line from your shoulders to your knees. Hold this position for a few seconds before lowering back down. The bridge helps correct anterior pelvic tilt by activating the posterior chain and encouraging proper alignment of the pelvis and spine.

Incorporating these exercises into your routine will not only help improve your posture but also enhance your overall strength and mobility, making it easier to maintain good posture throughout daily activities.

Ergonomic Techniques for Daily Life

In addition to exercises, making adjustments to your daily habits and environment can have a significant impact on posture. **Ergonomics**, the science of designing environments to fit the user, plays a crucial role in preventing poor posture and the associated health issues. By ensuring that your workspace, seating arrangements, and movement patterns support natural alignment, you can reduce the strain on your body and promote better posture.

If you spend long hours sitting, as many people do, investing in an **ergonomic chair** is essential. Look for a chair that supports the natural curve of your lower back, allowing you to sit with your feet flat on the ground and your knees at a 90-degree angle. Avoid slouching by sitting with your back pressed against the chair's backrest and using the armrests to support your shoulders in a relaxed position. If necessary, place a small cushion or rolled-up towel behind your lower back to maintain the natural lumbar curve.

For those who work at a desk, proper monitor placement is key. Your computer screen should be at **eye level**, so you don't have to tilt your head down or up to view it. This simple adjustment can help prevent forward head posture and reduce strain on the neck. Additionally, if you frequently use a smartphone or tablet, hold the device at eye level instead of looking down at it, which can exacerbate neck and upper back issues.

Another important ergonomic principle is to **take frequent breaks** to move and stretch. Sitting or standing in one position for extended periods can lead to muscle imbalances and stiffness. Aim to stand up and stretch every 30 to 60 minutes, incorporating gentle movements like shoulder rolls, neck stretches, or a short walk. These breaks help prevent the muscles from becoming fatigued and encourage better circulation, reducing the risk of posture-related pain.

If your job involves **lifting or carrying** heavy objects, practice proper lifting techniques to protect your back. Bend at the hips and knees, not the waist, and keep the object close to your body as you lift. Engaging your core and using your legs to lift, rather than your back, helps prevent strain and injury. For carrying objects, keep the load balanced and distribute weight evenly across both sides of the body to avoid overloading one side.

Standing desks can also be a helpful tool for improving posture, especially for those who work in sedentary jobs. **Alternating between sitting and standing** throughout the day allows you to shift your weight and engage different muscle groups, preventing the negative effects of prolonged sitting. When standing, make sure your weight is evenly distributed between both feet, and avoid locking your knees. If possible, use an anti-fatigue mat to reduce pressure on your feet and joints.

By incorporating these ergonomic adjustments into your daily life, you can create an environment that supports healthy posture and reduces the likelihood of discomfort or injury. Combined with posture-improving exercises, these strategies can help you maintain proper alignment and move through your day with greater ease and efficiency.

4.5 Tracking Progress

Tracking your progress is a crucial component of any fitness journey. It allows you to measure the effectiveness of your workout routine, adjust your approach as needed, and stay motivated as you work toward your goals. Whether you're aiming to improve strength, lose weight, or enhance your overall fitness, regularly monitoring your progress can help you stay on track and maintain accountability. The key is not just to focus on outcomes, but to track a variety of metrics that reflect the different aspects of your health and fitness journey.

Tools for Measuring Results

In today's fitness landscape, there are a variety of tools available to help you monitor your progress, from simple pen-and-paper logs to advanced wearable devices. Choosing the right tool depends on your personal preferences and the specific metrics you want to track. Regardless of the method you choose, consistency is key when measuring results, as it provides a clear picture of how your body is responding to your efforts.

One of the simplest ways to track progress is by **recording your workouts**. Keeping a workout log can provide valuable insights into your performance over time. For instance, tracking the weights you lift, the number of repetitions you perform, or the distance you run helps you see improvements in strength, endurance, and stamina. It also allows you to recognize patterns, such as when you hit a plateau or when certain workouts lead to better results. By reviewing your logs, you can make informed decisions about when to increase the intensity of your workouts or change your routine to keep your body challenged.

For those focused on body composition, **measuring key metrics** like weight, body fat percentage, and circumference measurements can offer tangible evidence of progress. While weight alone isn't always the best indicator of fitness, especially if you're building muscle, combining it with body fat percentage and measurements of your waist, hips, and other areas can give a more comprehensive view of your physical transformation. There are tools like calipers for body fat measurements, or for more precision, you might use a body composition scale or even a DEXA scan. These measurements help you see changes that might not be reflected on the scale alone, such as an increase in muscle mass or a decrease in fat.

In addition to these basic tools, **wearable fitness trackers** have become increasingly popular due to their ability to provide real-time data on your physical activity, heart rate, and even sleep patterns. Devices like fitness watches or smart bands can track how many steps you take, your daily calorie expenditure, and the intensity of your workouts. Some models even offer detailed analytics on your sleep, giving you a clearer picture of how well your body is recovering from exercise. Tracking your sleep and recovery is particularly important for maintaining long-term progress, as inadequate rest can negatively impact your workouts and overall performance.

For endurance athletes, tools like **GPS watches** and heart rate monitors can provide valuable data during workouts. These devices allow you to measure your pace, heart rate, and even elevation changes during runs, bike rides, or hikes. Monitoring your heart rate during exercise is particularly useful for ensuring you're working within the right intensity zone for your fitness goals—whether that means burning fat, building endurance, or improving cardiovascular health.

No matter which tools you use, it's important to remember that progress is not always linear. While numbers like weight, reps, or distances can be motivating, it's essential to look at the bigger picture. Improvement in overall fitness, mobility, and how you feel during and after workouts is just as important as the numbers on a chart.

How to Maintain Motivation

Maintaining motivation over the long term can be one of the biggest challenges in any fitness journey. Motivation often fluctuates, and it's normal to go through phases where you feel more or less driven. The key to maintaining progress is to develop strategies that keep you engaged, even when motivation wanes.

One of the most effective ways to stay motivated is by setting **specific and attainable goals**. Broad goals like "getting fit" or "losing weight" can feel overwhelming and vague, making it hard to stay focused. Instead, break these large goals down into smaller, more manageable targets. For example, you might set a goal to complete three workouts per week or to increase your deadlift by five pounds over the next month. By focusing on incremental progress, you create a sense of achievement that can keep you motivated over time. Each small success builds on the next, reinforcing the behavior and making it more likely that you will stick with your routine.

Another important factor in maintaining motivation is **variety**. Doing the same exercises or following the same routine day in and day out can lead to boredom, making it harder to stay consistent. Incorporating a variety of workouts, such as alternating between strength training, cardio, and flexibility exercises, can keep things fresh and exciting. Trying new activities, like yoga, swimming, or even a dance class, can also reignite your enthusiasm for fitness.

Keeping a **fitness journal** can also help you stay motivated by providing a place to reflect on your progress, set new goals, and record how you're feeling throughout your journey. In addition to logging your workouts, use the journal to note any challenges you've faced, how you overcame them, and what you're proud of each week. Over time, this can become a powerful tool for recognizing how far you've come, even on days when you feel like you're not making progress.

For many people, creating a **reward system** can provide additional motivation. Rewards don't have to be extravagant—something as simple as treating yourself to a new workout outfit, a healthy meal at your favorite restaurant, or a relaxing day off can be enough to keep you motivated. The key is to align your rewards with your fitness goals, ensuring they reinforce the positive behaviors you're working to establish.

It's also essential to recognize that **setbacks are a natural part of the process**. Whether it's missing a few workouts, not seeing progress as quickly as you'd like, or dealing with an injury, setbacks can be discouraging. The important thing is to not let them derail your efforts completely. Instead of viewing setbacks as failures, see them as opportunities to learn and adjust. Maybe you need more rest, a new routine, or a fresh perspective to keep moving forward.

Finally, surrounding yourself with **supportive people** can make a significant difference in maintaining motivation. Whether it's friends, family, or a fitness community, having a network of people who encourage you and hold you accountable can keep you on track, even when your motivation dips. Working out with a partner or joining a fitness group can provide the encouragement and accountability you need to push through tough times and celebrate successes together.

Sharing Progress with the Community

Sharing your progress with others can be a powerful motivator, and thanks to the rise of social media and fitness communities, it's easier than ever to connect with people who share your goals. Whether you post about your workouts on Instagram, join a Facebook fitness group, or track your progress on a fitness app, sharing your journey can provide a sense of accountability and support that keeps you moving forward.

Many people find that **documenting their progress publicly** motivates them to stay consistent, as it provides external validation and encouragement. Posting a progress photo, sharing a workout milestone, or talking about your goals with others can lead to positive feedback that reinforces your efforts. Social media platforms are filled with fitness communities where individuals share their successes, challenges, and tips, creating a space where people can support and inspire each other. Being part of such a community can make your fitness journey feel less isolating and more rewarding.

Beyond social media, **local fitness groups or classes** can offer a sense of camaraderie and belonging. Whether it's a group run, a yoga class, or a CrossFit community, working out with others provides a sense of connection that can enhance your experience. Many people find that they are more motivated to show up for workouts when they know they will see familiar faces and work toward common goals with others.

Sharing progress doesn't always have to be public. For some, keeping progress private but sharing with a trusted friend, coach, or trainer can provide similar benefits. These individuals can offer personalized feedback and encouragement, helping you stay accountable to your goals.

Incorporating progress-sharing into your fitness routine can be an effective way to stay engaged, maintain accountability, and receive support from others who understand the challenges and rewards of pursuing a fitness journey. Whether it's through social media, fitness apps, or personal relationships, finding ways to share your progress can make your fitness experience more enjoyable and sustainable over the long term.

Chapter 5: Resilience and Adaptation

5.1 Cold and Heat Exposure

Building resilience is about preparing the body and mind to endure and adapt to challenging conditions. One of the most effective ways to enhance physical and mental resilience is through controlled exposure to extreme environments, particularly cold and heat. This form of adaptation training not only strengthens the body but also improves metabolic efficiency, cardiovascular health, and mental fortitude. As we've explored in previous chapters, such as in our discussion on physical activity and metabolism, the human body is capable of remarkable adaptation when exposed to stressors. In this chapter, we will delve deeper into how controlled cold and heat exposure can act as beneficial stressors that enhance resilience and overall health.

Benefits of Adaptation Training

When the body is exposed to extreme temperatures, it is forced to adjust and adapt. This process, known as hormesis, involves exposing the body to small, manageable doses of stress to strengthen its response to future challenges. Just as we've seen with the benefits of regular exercise in Chapter 4, where physical activity serves as a positive stressor to build muscle and endurance, exposure to cold and heat also triggers adaptive responses that bolster resilience and health.

Cold exposure has been extensively studied for its ability to stimulate the nervous system, boost metabolism, and enhance immune function. When exposed to cold, the body works harder to maintain its core temperature, activating brown adipose tissue (brown fat), which burns calories to generate heat. This thermogenic process increases metabolic rate and supports fat loss. Cold exposure also improves circulation by constricting and then dilating blood vessels, which enhances vascular flexibility. In addition, short bouts of cold exposure can reduce inflammation, improve recovery from exercise, and enhance mental clarity.

Heat exposure, particularly through practices like **sauna use or heat therapy**, offers its own set of unique benefits. When the body is exposed to high temperatures, it triggers a cascade of physiological responses designed to protect and cool the body. Sweating, increased heart rate, and enhanced circulation all work together to maintain homeostasis.

Similar to the cardiovascular benefits of aerobic exercise discussed in Chapter 4, heat exposure improves heart health by stimulating blood flow and enhancing vascular function. Additionally, heat induces the production of heat shock proteins, which play a critical role in cellular repair and stress resistance. These proteins protect cells from damage, promote longevity, and aid in muscle recovery.

Both cold and heat exposure also offer profound mental health benefits. When you voluntarily expose yourself to discomfort, such as taking a cold shower or sitting in a sauna, you train your mind to handle stress more effectively. This mental resilience, or psychological hardiness, is essential for overcoming obstacles in life, as we'll discuss more in Chapter 5.3. The practice of enduring physical discomfort helps to improve mental toughness, reduce anxiety, and promote a sense of accomplishment and well-being.

Safe Exposure Techniques

While cold and heat exposure can offer numerous health benefits, it's important to approach these practices safely to avoid injury or adverse effects. Gradual adaptation is key, particularly for those new to this form of training. Much like the principle of progression in exercise routines, as outlined in Chapter 4.2, cold and heat exposure should start with manageable durations and intensities before gradually increasing the challenge.

For **cold exposure**, beginners might start with something as simple as ending a warm shower with 30 seconds of cold water. Over time, you can increase the duration of cold exposure, working up to full cold showers or even cold water immersion. When engaging in cold exposure, it's important to listen to your body. While discomfort is part of the process, pain or numbness can indicate that you've pushed too far. If you're taking ice baths or immersing in cold water, limit the exposure to 1-3 minutes initially, ensuring you're in a controlled environment where you can safely exit the water. Breathing exercises, such as those used in the Wim Hof Method, can also help you manage the physiological stress of cold exposure, keeping you calm and focused during the practice.

When it comes to **heat exposure**, such as using a sauna, it's equally important to start gradually. A typical sauna session might last anywhere from 10 to 20 minutes, but beginners should start with shorter durations to allow the body to acclimate. Drink plenty of water before and after to stay hydrated, as heat exposure leads to significant fluid loss through sweat. If you experience dizziness or light-headedness during heat exposure, it's a sign to exit and cool down. Over time, as your body adapts, you can extend your sessions and increase the temperature, reaping the cardiovascular and cellular benefits.

In both cold and heat exposure, it's crucial to avoid sudden, extreme changes in temperature. After cold exposure, gently warm the body with light movement or a warm drink, but avoid jumping into a hot shower immediately, as this can shock the system. Similarly, after heat exposure, allow your body to cool down gradually before taking a cold shower or stepping outside in cold weather.

Practical Examples and Guidelines

Incorporating cold and heat exposure into your routine can be simple, but consistency is key to maximizing the benefits. As we've seen with exercise routines, detailed in Chapter 4, regular practice leads to adaptation, whether it's in building strength or enhancing resilience to temperature extremes. Below are some practical examples of how to integrate cold and heat exposure into your daily life.

For cold exposure, start with **cold showers**, which are an accessible and easy way to begin adaptation training. After your regular warm shower, turn the water to cold for the last 30 seconds, focusing on deep, controlled breathing. As you get more comfortable, you can gradually extend the cold phase of your shower to 1-2 minutes or switch to full cold showers.

If you have access to a **cold plunge** or a body of cold water, you can use these for more intense cold exposure. Ice baths or cold water immersion can be particularly beneficial after intense exercise, aiding in recovery and reducing muscle soreness. Aim for short, controlled sessions of 1-3 minutes, building up over time as your tolerance improves.

For those interested in heat exposure, **sauna sessions** are one of the most effective methods. Aim to use a sauna 2-3 times per week, starting with short sessions of 10 minutes at a lower temperature, and gradually increasing both the duration and heat. Sauna use has been linked to improved cardiovascular health, increased longevity, and enhanced detoxification through sweat.

Another option for heat exposure is **hot yoga**, which combines the physical benefits of yoga with the added challenge of a heated environment. This practice helps improve flexibility, promotes detoxification, and encourages mental resilience as you learn to focus and breathe in challenging conditions.

For those without access to a sauna, simply spending time in a warm environment—whether through hot baths or heated rooms—can also provide some of the benefits. However, structured practices like sauna use or hot yoga are typically more effective in eliciting the physiological adaptations we've discussed.

As with any form of training, consistency is key. Cold and heat exposure should be seen as a regular part of your wellness routine, much like exercise or nutrition. By incorporating these practices into your life, you'll not only improve your physical resilience but also strengthen your mind, preparing you to handle stress and adversity in other areas of life.

Whether through cold water plunges or sauna sessions, the key to success is gradual adaptation, listening to your body, and maintaining a regular practice. These techniques offer profound benefits for both body and mind, building resilience that extends beyond physical challenges into daily life, work, and relationships.

5.2 Mind and Body Balance

In our pursuit of resilience and adaptation, the connection between mind and body plays a critical role. As discussed in earlier chapters, physical resilience is essential, but it's only one half of the equation. The mental and emotional aspects of health are just as important when striving for overall well-being and the ability to handle life's challenges. A strong mind-body connection ensures that we can not only endure physical stressors, such as those introduced in Chapter 5.1 through cold and heat exposure, but also adapt mentally and emotionally to adversity. To cultivate resilience, both aspects must be nurtured.

Importance of Mental Health

Mental health is the foundation upon which psychological resilience is built, and it influences every facet of life, including physical health. We've seen in Chapter 4 how exercise can positively impact mental health by releasing endorphins, improving sleep quality, and reducing anxiety. Physical activity is a powerful tool, but it's important to recognize that the mind needs its own strategies for care and balance, independent of physical efforts.

When mental health suffers, it affects not only emotional well-being but also physical health. Chronic stress, for instance, has been linked to numerous physical ailments, including heart disease, obesity, and metabolic dysfunction. Prolonged stress can lead to increased cortisol levels, which disrupts sleep, hampers digestion, and weakens the immune system. Over time, these effects can contribute to a cycle of declining health that is difficult to reverse without addressing the root mental causes.

Good mental health, on the other hand, acts as a buffer against life's inevitable challenges. It promotes a sense of calm and emotional stability, even in the face of stress. People who take active steps to care for their mental health, whether through mindfulness, therapy, or self-care practices, are more likely to maintain balance during difficult times. Just as you build physical strength and resilience through training and adaptation, the mind can be strengthened through consistent mental health practices.

Mental health is especially important in today's fast-paced, high-pressure world. Anxiety, depression, and stress-related disorders are more common than ever, and neglecting mental well-being can have serious consequences. Addressing mental health proactively, much like we focus on preventing physical illness, is key to living a balanced life. The mind and body must work together to create resilience, and neglecting one will inevitably weaken the other.

Psychological Resilience Techniques

Building psychological resilience is an intentional process that involves training the mind to adapt to stress, uncertainty, and adversity. Just as we discussed the gradual adaptation process for physical stressors in Chapter 5.1, psychological resilience is developed by consistently facing mental challenges with effective coping strategies. Resilience doesn't mean avoiding stress; instead, it means handling stress in a way that prevents it from overwhelming you.

One of the most well-researched and effective methods for developing psychological resilience is **mindfulness**. Mindfulness is the practice of staying present in the moment without judgment. It allows individuals to observe their thoughts and emotions without becoming entangled in them. This practice helps to regulate the nervous system, calm the mind, and reduce the feelings of anxiety or overwhelm that can arise during stressful situations.

Mindfulness can be as simple as taking a few minutes each day to focus on your breathing. Breathing exercises, like **deep diaphragmatic breathing** or **box breathing**, are powerful tools for managing the body's response to stress. When we engage in these slow, controlled breathing patterns, we activate the parasympathetic nervous system, which helps reduce the production of cortisol and brings the body into a more relaxed state. By doing this regularly, you train your body and mind to respond more calmly to stressors, improving overall resilience.

Another key technique is **cognitive reframing**. This involves changing the way you perceive and interpret events. Cognitive reframing helps you shift from a negative or defeatist mindset to one that is more constructive and solution-focused. For instance, rather than viewing a challenge as insurmountable, cognitive reframing encourages you to see it as an opportunity for growth or learning. This mindset shift reduces the emotional weight of difficult situations and promotes a more resilient outlook.

Incorporating **gratitude practices** into your daily life is another powerful way to bolster psychological resilience. Gratitude has been shown to improve mental health by fostering a positive outlook, even in challenging times. As we will further explore in Chapter 8.3, regularly reflecting on what you are grateful for—whether it's big or small—helps shift your focus away from stressors and towards the positives in your life. This daily practice rewires the brain to notice the good, cultivating emotional strength over time.

Self-compassion is equally important when building resilience. Often, when faced with failure or setbacks, people tend to be overly critical of themselves, which can erode mental health. Self-compassion involves treating yourself with the same kindness and understanding that you would extend to a friend. Instead of berating yourself for not handling a situation perfectly, self-compassion allows you to acknowledge your humanity, learn from the experience, and move forward without the burden of guilt or shame.

Another resilience-building tool is **psychological flexibility**. This refers to the ability to adapt to changing circumstances and remain open to new ideas and experiences. People with high psychological flexibility can shift their mindset and behaviors to better cope with stress and uncertainty. They are able to focus on what they can control, rather than becoming paralyzed by factors beyond their influence. By practicing flexibility in your thinking, you create more mental space to navigate challenges creatively and with less emotional distress.

Creating a Positive Mindset

A positive mindset is essential for fostering psychological resilience and maintaining mental health. This does not mean ignoring the difficulties in life or pretending that everything is always fine. Rather, a positive mindset is about approaching challenges with an optimistic and constructive attitude, believing that you can overcome obstacles and learn from adversity.

One way to cultivate a positive mindset is through **positive self-talk**. The language you use when speaking to yourself has a direct impact on your confidence and resilience. Negative self-talk—such as "I'll never succeed" or "I'm not good enough"—undermines your efforts and reinforces feelings of helplessness. Conversely, positive self-talk—such as "I'm capable of handling this" or "I've overcome challenges before"—boosts your confidence and helps you stay focused on finding solutions.

Visualization is another effective technique for creating a positive mindset. This involves mentally rehearsing success before it happens, helping you to feel more prepared and confident when facing challenges. Athletes often use visualization techniques before competitions, but this tool can be applied to any situation where you want to perform at your best. By visualizing yourself successfully navigating a difficult situation, you reduce anxiety and build mental resilience.

Goal setting, as discussed in Chapter 4.2, plays a significant role in maintaining a positive mindset as well. Clear, achievable goals provide structure and purpose, giving you something to work toward even in the face of adversity. Setting small, attainable goals allows you to experience regular success, which in turn reinforces a positive outlook. It's important to focus on progress rather than perfection, celebrating each milestone as a step forward.

In addition to mental techniques, **environmental factors** can greatly influence your mindset. Surrounding yourself with positive influences—whether that's through supportive relationships, inspirational media, or uplifting activities—reinforces a mindset of growth and resilience. We will explore this concept further in Chapter 5.5, where we discuss the importance of community and support systems. Engaging with people who encourage you and who share your values can greatly enhance your ability to maintain a positive mindset, even in challenging times.

In the end, creating a positive mindset is not about forcing positivity in every situation. It's about recognizing the power you have to influence your thoughts, emotions, and actions. By practicing self-compassion, using cognitive reframing techniques, and cultivating gratitude, you build a foundation for psychological resilience that helps you navigate life's challenges with greater ease. This balance between mind and body fosters a deeper sense of well-being and supports your ability to adapt and thrive in a constantly changing world.

5.3 Overcoming Obstacles

Life is full of obstacles, both large and small, and our ability to face these challenges defines much of our personal and professional success. Overcoming obstacles requires not just physical resilience, as we discussed in Chapter 5.1, but also mental and emotional strength. Resilience isn't about avoiding difficulties but about learning how to navigate them effectively. In this section, we will explore strategies for facing challenges, the crucial role of perseverance, and how social support systems act as vital safety nets during times of difficulty.

Strategies for Facing Challenges

Every obstacle presents a unique set of challenges, but effective strategies for overcoming them share common principles. One of the most important factors in overcoming difficulties is **mindset**. As discussed in Chapter 5.2, cultivating a positive and resilient mindset plays a significant role in how you approach challenges. When you believe in your ability to navigate hardships, you're more likely to find solutions and remain focused on your goals.

Breaking down problems into manageable parts is a crucial strategy for tackling obstacles. Large challenges can seem overwhelming, leading to paralysis and inaction. However, by dividing the issue into smaller, more manageable steps, you can reduce the feeling of being overwhelmed. For example, if you're facing a significant professional setback, start by identifying the immediate actions you can take—whether that's reassessing your goals, seeking feedback, or learning a new skill. Tackling one small aspect at a time builds momentum, gradually leading to a solution.

Another key approach is **flexibility and adaptability**. Many obstacles arise from unexpected changes, and rigidly adhering to one course of action can limit your ability to overcome them. As we discussed in Chapter 5.2 with psychological flexibility, the ability to adapt to new circumstances is essential for resilience. Whether it's adjusting a business strategy, changing a personal plan, or rethinking your approach to a health goal, being open to new ideas and solutions is crucial.

Problem-solving skills are also essential in overcoming obstacles. Critical thinking, creativity, and resourcefulness enable you to explore all possible solutions rather than getting stuck on what isn't working. When facing a challenge, ask yourself, "What are my options?" or "What haven't I considered yet?" By shifting your focus to what can be done instead of what can't, you empower yourself to find new pathways to success.

In addition, **emotional regulation** is key when dealing with challenges. Stress and anxiety can cloud judgment, making it difficult to think clearly or make good decisions. Techniques like mindfulness, as mentioned in Chapter 5.2, can help you stay calm and focused even when faced with intense pressure. Taking time to step back, breathe, and assess the situation with a clear mind often leads to more effective problem-solving and better outcomes.

Finally, **acceptance** is an important yet often overlooked strategy. Not all challenges are fully within our control, and recognizing what you can't change can be just as important as focusing on what you can. Acceptance doesn't mean giving up; it means acknowledging reality and working within it, rather than resisting it. This shift in perspective can help free up mental energy to focus on actionable solutions.

The Importance of Perseverance

Perseverance is the backbone of overcoming obstacles. It's not enough to simply face challenges—you must continue to push forward, even when progress is slow or setbacks occur. As we've seen in previous chapters, success in both mental and physical health often comes from consistent effort over time. Perseverance ensures that you stay committed to your goals, even when immediate results are not visible.

One of the key aspects of perseverance is the ability to **reframe setbacks as opportunities for growth**. Instead of viewing failure as an endpoint, see it as part of the process. In Chapter 5.2, we discussed the power of cognitive reframing—using setbacks as learning experiences can help you maintain a positive outlook and stay motivated. Each time you persevere through a challenge, you strengthen your resilience and increase your capacity to handle future obstacles.

Perseverance also requires **patience**. Many obstacles, particularly those related to long-term goals, cannot be overcome quickly. Whether you're working toward a fitness goal, career advancement, or personal development, progress often happens incrementally. As we discussed in Chapter 4.5, tracking progress over time can help you stay focused and motivated, even when the pace feels slow. Remember that consistency is more important than intensity; steady, regular effort often leads to greater success than short bursts of intense effort followed by burnout.

Another aspect of perseverance is **self-discipline**. This involves sticking to your goals even when it's uncomfortable or when immediate gratification is not possible. It's about making the tough choices that align with your long-term objectives, even when it would be easier to give up or take a shortcut. Developing self-discipline is crucial for overcoming obstacles because it ensures that you stay on track, even in the face of temptations or distractions.

Moreover, perseverance fosters **resilience** through repeated exposure to difficulty. Each time you face a challenge and push through, you build emotional and mental toughness. This cumulative process creates a strong foundation that helps you handle increasingly difficult situations. Like building muscle through regular exercise, perseverance strengthens your ability to endure hardship and bounce back from setbacks.

Social Support and Safety Nets

While individual perseverance is vital, overcoming obstacles is not something that should be done entirely alone. As we discussed in Chapter 5.2, surrounding yourself with positive influences plays a crucial role in maintaining a healthy mindset. In the same way, having a strong social support system can significantly ease the burden of facing challenges.

Social support comes in many forms—family, friends, mentors, colleagues, or even online communities. These people can provide emotional encouragement, practical advice, and, in some cases, direct assistance. When you're facing a difficult situation, talking to someone who understands or has been through something similar can provide new perspectives and remind you that you're not alone. Whether it's a simple conversation or a more structured form of support, such as counseling, having others to rely on makes challenges feel less daunting.

Support systems also serve as **safety nets** during periods of high stress or when things don't go as planned. For example, if you're struggling with a work-related issue, a trusted mentor might offer advice or help you navigate the situation more effectively. Similarly, friends and family can provide emotional support during personal hardships, offering encouragement and a listening ear when needed most.

Beyond immediate social connections, **formal support networks** such as professional organizations, support groups, or therapy can offer structured assistance for specific challenges. As we will further explore in Chapter 5.5, engaging in support groups or communities—whether in person or online—can create a sense of belonging and provide resources that help you overcome personal and professional obstacles. These networks often provide collective wisdom and shared experiences, making it easier to find solutions or simply cope with the emotional toll of facing difficulties.

It's also important to remember that asking for help is a sign of strength, not weakness. Many people hesitate to reach out because they don't want to burden others or feel that they should be able to handle challenges on their own. However, leveraging social support can provide the assistance you need to persevere through tough times, and in turn, you can be a source of support for others when they face their own obstacles.

Furthermore, **building meaningful relationships** creates a reciprocal safety net. When you invest time and energy in your social connections, you strengthen the bonds that will support you during tough times. This sense of community, whether through friends, family, or professional networks, provides a foundation of security that allows you to take risks, face challenges, and know that you have people who will back you up if things don't go as planned.

Incorporating **social support** into your strategy for overcoming obstacles not only helps you manage immediate challenges but also promotes long-term resilience. The feeling of connectedness and belonging that comes from a strong support system can boost mental health, provide emotional relief, and enhance your overall ability to face life's difficulties.

In summary, overcoming obstacles requires a multifaceted approach that includes effective problem-solving strategies, perseverance, and strong social support. By cultivating resilience, building mental strength, and maintaining a network of people who can help you along the way, you increase your chances of not just overcoming obstacles but thriving in the face of adversity.

5.4 Prevention and Preparedness for Illness

Prevention and preparedness are critical components of maintaining long-term health, as they allow individuals to take control of their well-being before illness strikes. We've discussed how physical and mental resilience contribute to overall health in earlier chapters, such as the benefits of exercise, nutrition, and stress management (Chapter 4 and Chapter 5). In this section, we'll dive deeper into recognizing early warning signs of illness, adopting preventive strategies that protect your health, and creating a personal emergency plan to ensure you're ready to respond when necessary.

How to Recognize Warning Signs

The human body is adept at signaling when something is wrong, but the challenge lies in recognizing these early signs before they escalate into more serious health problems. As we explored in Chapter 1.2, tracking biomarkers is an effective way to assess your metabolic health. Similarly, paying close attention to how your body feels and functions daily allows you to detect the early onset of illness.

Early warning signs of illness can range from subtle changes in energy levels or mood to more noticeable physical symptoms. **Fatigue** is one of the most common early indicators that something is wrong. While occasional tiredness can result from a busy lifestyle, persistent fatigue—especially if it's not alleviated by rest—could indicate underlying conditions such as anemia, hypothyroidism, or even mental health issues like depression. Fatigue can also be linked to chronic infections or inflammatory diseases, meaning that paying attention to ongoing tiredness is essential for early intervention.

Unexplained weight loss or gain is another potential red flag. While fluctuations in weight are normal, sudden and unexplained changes may suggest an underlying issue. For example, rapid weight loss without a change in diet or exercise could indicate conditions such as hyperthyroidism, diabetes, or cancer. On the other hand, weight gain, particularly when accompanied by swelling in the extremities or abdomen, may point to heart disease, kidney problems, or hormonal imbalances. Regularly monitoring your weight, along with other biomarkers, can help catch these early warning signs.

Digestive issues, such as persistent bloating, diarrhea, constipation, or heartburn, can also be a sign of an underlying health problem. Gastrointestinal disturbances might indicate food intolerances, infections, or more serious conditions like irritable bowel syndrome (IBS), celiac disease, or even colon cancer. While occasional digestive upset is normal, chronic or severe symptoms should prompt a visit to a healthcare professional.

Equally important are **mental health changes**, as the mind and body are closely interconnected. An increase in irritability, anxiety, or feelings of depression may signal not just a psychological issue, but also a physical one. For instance, vitamin D deficiency, thyroid problems, or chronic inflammation have all been linked to mood disorders. As noted in Chapter 5.2, mental health warning signs often present themselves in subtle ways, and it's important to address these signals as part of an overall health strategy.

Other physical symptoms, such as **chronic pain**, can also serve as early indicators of illness. Persistent back pain, headaches, or joint pain may be the result of stress, injury, or an underlying condition such as arthritis, fibromyalgia, or nerve disorders. Chronic pain should never be ignored, as it often signals that something is amiss within the body.

Finally, **changes in the skin**—such as new rashes, persistent itching, changes in moles, or unexplained bruising—can serve as early indicators of internal issues. The skin is often referred to as a window into overall health, and sudden changes may point to conditions such as allergies, liver disease, or even skin cancer.

The key to recognizing early warning signs is **self-awareness**. By staying attuned to how your body normally feels and functions, you can quickly identify changes that may warrant medical attention. Additionally, routine check-ups and preventive screenings, as discussed in Chapter 6, can help catch issues before they progress into more serious problems.

Preventive Strategies to Adopt

Prevention is about taking proactive steps to reduce the likelihood of illness and promoting long-term health. Just as we've emphasized the importance of consistency in diet and exercise throughout this book, preventive health strategies should be part of your everyday routine.

Nutrition is one of the most powerful tools in illness prevention. As explored in Chapter 2, a balanced diet rich in essential nutrients helps support the immune system, reduce inflammation, and prevent the development of chronic conditions like heart disease, diabetes, and certain cancers. For instance, eating foods high in antioxidants, such as fruits and vegetables, helps combat oxidative stress, which can damage cells and contribute to disease. Omega-3 fatty acids, found in fish like salmon or plant sources like flaxseeds, reduce inflammation and improve heart health. Additionally, a diet rich in **fiber** promotes gut health, which is closely linked to immune function. High-fiber foods, such as whole grains, legumes, and leafy greens, not only improve digestion but also help regulate blood sugar and lower cholesterol levels.

Hydration is another essential aspect of prevention. Staying hydrated supports bodily functions such as digestion, nutrient absorption, and temperature regulation. Dehydration can lead to fatigue, impaired cognitive function, and increased susceptibility to illness. Water is crucial for flushing out toxins, keeping the skin healthy, and maintaining proper blood circulation. Drinking enough water daily—typically around 8 glasses for most adults, though individual needs vary—ensures that your body can function at its best.

Physical activity is perhaps one of the most important preventive measures you can take. Regular exercise, as detailed in Chapter 4, strengthens the heart, improves lung capacity, and enhances immune function. Physical activity helps regulate body weight, reduces the risk of developing metabolic diseases like diabetes, and lowers blood pressure. It also promotes the release of endorphins, improving mental health and reducing stress, which, as discussed in Chapter 5.2, is essential for overall well-being.

Exercise doesn't have to be intense to be effective. Even moderate activities like walking, cycling, or swimming can help reduce inflammation, improve circulation, and boost immune response. The key is to incorporate movement into your daily routine consistently, whether through structured workouts or daily habits like walking more or taking the stairs.

Sleep is another cornerstone of preventive health, as outlined in Chapter 3. Poor sleep not only weakens the immune system but also increases the risk of developing chronic conditions like heart disease, diabetes, and obesity. Getting adequate sleep each night (generally 7-9 hours for most adults) allows the body to repair itself, reduce inflammation, and regulate hormones. To support good sleep hygiene, maintain a regular sleep schedule, create a relaxing bedtime routine, and keep your sleeping environment free from distractions like bright lights or electronic devices.

Managing stress is crucial for illness prevention, as chronic stress has been linked to a wide range of health problems, including heart disease, depression, and autoimmune conditions. Mindfulness, meditation, and deep breathing exercises can help reduce the physical impact of stress on the body. Chapter 5.2 discussed the importance of mental resilience, and stress management plays a large part in maintaining both mental and physical health. Taking regular breaks, engaging in hobbies, and spending time with loved ones are all effective strategies for keeping stress in check.

Preventive care also includes **vaccinations and screenings**. Vaccines help protect against diseases like the flu, pneumonia, and certain cancers (such as the HPV vaccine). Regular health screenings, including cholesterol checks, blood pressure monitoring, and cancer screenings (such as mammograms or colonoscopies), catch potential issues early, allowing for timely treatment.

Creating a Personal Emergency Plan

While preventive strategies can go a long way in protecting your health, it's important to be prepared for unexpected health emergencies. As we discussed in Chapter 4.5, tracking progress helps you stay on top of your health goals. Similarly, creating a personal emergency plan ensures you are prepared to act quickly and effectively when faced with a health crisis.

The first step in creating a personal emergency plan is **understanding your unique health risks**. For example, if you have a family history of heart disease, diabetes, or other chronic conditions, your emergency plan should account for these specific risks. Similarly, if you have known allergies or a condition that requires immediate treatment (such as asthma), your plan should outline steps for managing an acute episode. This might include knowing the signs of an impending asthma attack or an allergic reaction and having the necessary medications or tools (such as an inhaler or EpiPen) readily available.

Your emergency plan should also include **detailed medical information**. Keep a record of your current medications, medical history, and any allergies you may have. Make sure this information is easily accessible in case of emergency, either stored in a physical document or on a secure app that can be quickly retrieved.

Another critical aspect of emergency preparedness is knowing where to seek care. Identify the nearest **emergency room or urgent care center**, and ensure that you're aware of any specific facilities that can address your health needs (such as cardiac specialists or stroke centers). If you travel frequently, be aware of where local healthcare facilities are located in the areas you visit. Knowing where to go in an emergency ensures that you can receive care promptly, which is often the key to better outcomes in serious situations.

For those with chronic conditions, creating an **action plan for acute symptoms or flare-ups** is crucial. This plan should outline exactly what to do if your condition worsens or you experience new symptoms. For instance, if you have diabetes, your plan might include steps to take if your blood sugar drops or spikes unexpectedly. Having a clear plan in place reduces confusion and panic in the moment, allowing for swift and appropriate action.

Additionally, ensure that you have designated **emergency contacts** who are familiar with your medical history and know how to assist you in a crisis. This could be a family member, friend, or caregiver. Communicate your emergency plan to them

5.5 The Importance of a Supportive Community

A supportive community plays a vital role in promoting physical, mental, and emotional well-being. Throughout this book, we've discussed various strategies for maintaining health and resilience, from regular exercise to stress management. But it's important to remember that humans are inherently social beings, and our connections with others can greatly influence our overall health. Whether it's through meaningful relationships, engagement in support groups, or leveraging local and online resources, community support is an indispensable element of a balanced and resilient life.

Building Meaningful Relationships

The foundation of a supportive community lies in **building meaningful relationships**. These connections can take many forms, including friendships, family bonds, mentorships, and professional networks. Meaningful relationships provide emotional support, a sense of belonging, and opportunities for growth. In Chapter 5.2, we explored how mental resilience is strengthened through emotional balance and positive thinking, and meaningful relationships are crucial to maintaining that balance.

A strong network of relationships offers a **sense of security**. Knowing that you have people who care about you and who are willing to listen and offer guidance when needed creates a foundation of emotional stability. In times of stress or difficulty, having someone to turn to can ease the burden of challenges and help you process your emotions in a healthy way. Conversely, the absence of meaningful relationships can contribute to feelings of isolation, anxiety, and depression, which, over time, can negatively impact both mental and physical health.

To build and maintain these meaningful connections, it's important to cultivate **open communication** and mutual trust. Relationships thrive on the ability to be honest and vulnerable with one another. Whether you're discussing personal challenges, sharing successes, or simply enjoying each other's company, the ability to connect on a deeper level fosters emotional intimacy, which is a key factor in mental well-being.

Meaningful relationships also offer **opportunities for growth**. Having people in your life who challenge you to think differently, encourage you to pursue your goals, and hold you accountable can significantly impact your personal development. Just as a workout partner might push you to reach new levels of fitness (as discussed in Chapter 4), a strong emotional connection can inspire you to achieve mental and emotional growth. This support can help you navigate challenges more effectively, whether in your personal life or professional endeavors.

Additionally, meaningful relationships create a **feedback loop of positivity**. When you offer support and encouragement to others, you not only strengthen the relationship, but you also reinforce your own sense of purpose and fulfillment. Helping others can boost your self-esteem, create a greater sense of empathy, and even reduce stress, all of which contribute to long-term resilience.

To nurture these relationships, it's important to **prioritize time for connection**. In our busy, fast-paced world, it's easy to neglect personal relationships in favor of professional responsibilities or individual pursuits. However, making time for loved ones, whether through regular phone calls, shared meals, or engaging in activities together, is crucial for maintaining strong bonds. Relationships require effort, and consistently investing in them ensures that they remain a source of support and joy.

How to Engage in Support Groups

While building personal relationships is essential, sometimes challenges arise that require a different kind of support. Engaging in **support groups** can provide additional emotional and practical help, especially when dealing with specific issues such as illness, grief, addiction, or mental health concerns. Support groups offer a structured environment where individuals facing similar challenges can share experiences, provide advice, and offer encouragement.

Support groups can be **formal or informal**. Formal support groups are often led by professionals, such as therapists or counselors, and follow a structured format. These groups may focus on specific issues like depression, anxiety, cancer recovery, or caregiving. The structure of these groups provides a safe space where individuals can express their feelings, learn coping strategies, and receive guidance from both professionals and peers. By connecting with others who are experiencing similar struggles, participants can gain valuable insights and emotional support that might not be available in their immediate social circles.

Informal support groups, on the other hand, are often peer-led and may not follow a strict structure. These groups can range from online forums to local meetups where people with shared interests or challenges come together to talk and offer support. For example, a local group for new parents might meet to discuss the challenges of raising children, share parenting tips, and provide a space for emotional support. These groups may not have a professional facilitator, but they offer an opportunity for connection and community building.

Engaging in support groups can offer several benefits. First, they provide **validation and understanding**. When dealing with a personal challenge, it's easy to feel isolated or misunderstood, especially if those around you haven't experienced the same issues. In a support group, members share their own stories and struggles, which can make participants feel less alone in their experience. Hearing how others have overcome similar challenges can also provide hope and inspiration.

Second, support groups often provide **practical advice**. In many cases, group members can offer suggestions for coping mechanisms, treatment options, or other resources that can be helpful in managing specific issues. Whether it's advice on navigating a medical condition, dealing with grief, or managing stress, the collective wisdom of the group can be a valuable resource.

To engage in a support group, the first step is to **identify what kind of support you need**. For example, if you're dealing with a specific health condition, look for groups that focus on that particular issue. If you're seeking emotional support for mental health concerns, a group that focuses on anxiety or depression might be more appropriate. Once you've identified the right group, make a commitment to attend regularly. Consistent participation helps build trust with other members and allows you to fully engage with the group's process.

In many cases, you can find support groups through **local community centers, hospitals, or counseling clinics**. These organizations often offer group sessions for people dealing with health issues, mental health challenges, or other life stressors. Additionally, online support groups are an excellent resource for those who prefer virtual engagement or are unable to attend in person.

Local and Online Resources for Wellbeing

In today's interconnected world, both **local and online resources** can offer valuable support for maintaining mental and physical health. These resources provide access to information, tools, and communities that can enhance your overall well-being.

Local resources often include wellness centers, gyms, community programs, and healthcare facilities. Many cities have local organizations dedicated to promoting physical and mental health through fitness classes, yoga, meditation, nutrition workshops, and mental health seminars. These programs offer not only the chance to improve personal well-being but also the opportunity to connect with others who share similar goals. For example, a local fitness class can serve as both a physical health resource and a way to build social connections with like-minded individuals. Likewise, community centers often provide access to affordable or free mental health services, such as counseling or stress management workshops.

Local healthcare providers, such as **therapists, nutritionists, or wellness coaches**, can also play a crucial role in your health journey. These professionals offer tailored guidance, support, and expertise, helping you navigate personal health challenges with personalized care. Establishing regular contact with trusted healthcare providers ensures that you have the necessary tools to prevent illness and manage stress, as discussed in Chapter 5.4.

In addition to local resources, the **online world** provides a wealth of tools for maintaining well-being. Whether through fitness apps, mental health platforms, or social media communities, the internet offers access to information and support that was previously unavailable. For example, mental health apps such as **Headspace** or **Calm** offer guided meditation, mindfulness exercises, and stress-relief techniques, allowing users to practice mental health care from the comfort of their homes. These platforms are accessible to everyone, making it easier to prioritize mental health regardless of location or schedule.

Online communities and forums, such as **Reddit** or **Facebook groups**, provide spaces where individuals can connect with others facing similar challenges or pursuing similar goals. Whether you're looking for advice on health and fitness, managing chronic illness, or improving mental health, these online platforms allow for peer-to-peer support and sharing of resources. In particular, for people in rural areas or those with limited access to local resources, online communities can provide a vital sense of connection and support.

Another valuable online resource is **telemedicine**, which has become increasingly popular in recent years. Telemedicine allows you to consult with healthcare professionals remotely, ensuring that you can access care even if you're unable to visit a clinic in person. This technology is especially useful for those managing chronic conditions, mental health care, or those with mobility challenges. It offers a convenient and accessible way to stay on top of your health without sacrificing time or quality of care.

By integrating both local and online resources into your wellness routine, you can create a comprehensive support system that promotes long-term health and resilience. These resources, combined with the meaningful relationships and support groups discussed earlier, create a robust network that supports your mental, emotional, and physical well-being.

Chapter 6: Navigating the Healthcare System

Navigating the healthcare system can be a daunting and often overwhelming task, especially when faced with a medical issue or when seeking preventative care. However, understanding the structure of the healthcare system, knowing the types of professionals you might encounter, and becoming aware of your patient rights can empower you to make informed decisions about your health. In this chapter, we will explore how to effectively engage with the healthcare system, how to choose the right specialist for your needs, and why knowing your rights as a patient is essential for receiving quality care.

6.1 Understanding the Healthcare System

The healthcare system can seem complex, with numerous layers, types of services, and different paths depending on your needs. Whether you're visiting a primary care physician, seeking specialist treatment, or undergoing surgery, the healthcare system is designed to provide comprehensive care. However, navigating this system requires a basic understanding of its structure, which varies from country to country but generally shares some common principles.

In most systems, healthcare is organized into **primary, secondary, and tertiary care**. Primary care is the first point of contact for most patients and includes general practitioners (GPs), family doctors, and pediatricians. These providers manage common health issues, offer preventive care, and refer patients to specialists if necessary. Secondary care includes specialized medical services provided by experts such as cardiologists, dermatologists, and orthopedists. Tertiary care involves highly specialized treatment, often in hospitals or specialized centers, and may include procedures like surgeries or treatment for severe illnesses.

Understanding this hierarchy helps when determining what type of care you need. For example, if you have a general health concern, such as fatigue or frequent headaches, your primary care provider (PCP) is usually the best place to start. They can assess your symptoms, provide basic treatments, and refer you to a specialist if needed. However, if you already know that you require specialized care—such as ongoing management of a chronic condition or surgery—you may need to enter the healthcare system at the secondary or tertiary level.

It's also important to understand the **logistics** of accessing healthcare. Many healthcare systems require referrals from primary care doctors before seeing a specialist, especially in systems like the National Health Service (NHS) in the UK or managed care systems in the US. In some cases, skipping this step could result in higher costs or delayed care. On the other hand, private healthcare systems or insurance plans might allow for more direct access to specialists, though this often depends on the specifics of your health insurance coverage.

Types of Health Professionals

One of the keys to navigating the healthcare system effectively is understanding the different types of health professionals you might encounter and what roles they play. Each type of healthcare provider has a specific area of expertise, and knowing whom to consult can save time, reduce frustration, and ensure you receive the right kind of care.

●**Primary Care Physicians (PCPs)**: As mentioned earlier, PCPs are often the first point of contact for patients. They handle routine check-ups, vaccinations, and minor illnesses and provide preventive care. PCPs may include general practitioners, family doctors, and pediatricians, who cater to children's health needs.

●**Nurse Practitioners (NPs)** and **Physician Assistants (PAs)**: These professionals can often provide many of the same services as doctors, including diagnosing and treating illnesses, prescribing medications, and providing preventive care. NPs and PAs are often part of a primary care team and can be a more accessible option in certain healthcare settings.

●**Specialists**: Specialists are doctors who have completed additional training in a specific area of medicine. Common specialists include cardiologists (heart), endocrinologists (hormones and diabetes), dermatologists (skin), and neurologists (brain and nervous system). Specialists focus on diagnosing and treating specific conditions and often work in secondary or tertiary care.

●**Surgeons**: Surgeons specialize in performing operations, ranging from routine procedures like appendectomies to more complex surgeries such as heart bypasses. They are typically involved in tertiary care.

●**Therapists**: Physical, occupational, and speech therapists help patients recover from injuries, surgeries, or illnesses that impact mobility, daily functioning, or communication. They work closely with patients to improve their quality of life through rehabilitation.

●**Mental Health Professionals**: These include psychiatrists, psychologists, counselors, and social workers who specialize in treating mental health conditions such as depression, anxiety, and bipolar disorder. Psychiatrists can prescribe medications, while psychologists and counselors typically focus on therapy and behavioral interventions.

●**Pharmacists**: Pharmacists are medication experts who ensure that patients receive the correct prescriptions and understand how to take their medications safely. They can provide guidance on potential side effects and how different drugs interact with each other.

●**Registered Nurses (RNs) and Licensed Practical Nurses (LPNs)**: Nurses provide critical care in many settings, including hospitals, clinics, and community health centers. RNs typically have more advanced training and handle complex patient needs, while LPNs provide basic nursing care under the supervision of RNs or doctors.

Knowing the roles of these professionals can help you make more informed decisions about who to consult depending on your healthcare needs. For example, if you're managing a chronic illness like diabetes, you might see both an endocrinologist for specialized care and a PCP for regular check-ups.

How to Choose the Right Specialist

Choosing the right specialist can be daunting, especially when you're dealing with a specific health issue that requires expert attention. The first step in finding the right specialist is often obtaining a referral from your PCP, who can assess your condition and recommend the appropriate specialist.

However, there are additional steps you can take to ensure you select the best specialist for your needs:

1.   **Research the Specialist's Credentials**: When choosing a specialist, it's important to verify their credentials. Board certification in their specialty is a key indicator that the doctor has the necessary training and expertise. You can typically find information about a doctor's credentials on healthcare websites, hospital profiles, or through

professional boards like the American Medical Association (AMA) or the General Medical Council (GMC) in the UK.

2. **Consider Experience**: Experience matters, especially for complex or rare conditions. If you require surgery or treatment for a specific illness, look for specialists with extensive experience in managing that condition. Ask how many procedures they've performed or how long they've been treating patients with your specific health issue.

3. **Read Reviews and Seek Referrals**: Online reviews and testimonials from other patients can provide insights into the specialist's communication style, bedside manner, and overall quality of care. Additionally, ask your primary care doctor, friends, or family members if they have personal recommendations.

4. **Check Insurance Coverage**: Before choosing a specialist, ensure that they are covered under your insurance plan. Out-of-network care can result in higher out-of-pocket costs, so it's essential to verify coverage in advance. Your insurance provider can usually provide a list of covered specialists within your network.

5. **Schedule a Consultation**: Meeting with a specialist before committing to treatment allows you to assess whether they are the right fit for you. During the consultation, ask questions about their approach to treatment, the options available, and any concerns you may have. Pay attention to how well the specialist listens and whether they explain things clearly.

6. **Evaluate Accessibility**: Consider practical factors such as the location of the specialist's office, availability of appointments, and whether they offer telemedicine services. Specialists with long wait times or inaccessible locations may not be the best option if you need timely care.

Patient Rights

Understanding your **patient rights** is critical for ensuring that you receive high-quality care and are treated fairly throughout your healthcare journey. These rights are designed to protect you as a patient and give you control over your healthcare decisions.

Key patient rights include:

●**Informed Consent**: Before any treatment or procedure, healthcare providers must explain the risks, benefits, and alternatives, allowing you to make an informed decision.

You have the right to ask questions and fully understand what's being proposed before consenting to treatment.

●**Privacy and Confidentiality**: Under laws like HIPAA (Health Insurance Portability and Accountability Act) in the US or GDPR (General Data Protection Regulation) in Europe, your personal health information must be kept private. Providers are required to protect your medical records and can only share them with authorized individuals.

●**Access to Care**: You have the right to access necessary medical care, regardless of personal characteristics such as race, gender, or disability. If you feel that you've been denied care or discriminated against, it's important to speak up or file a complaint with the relevant health authority.

●**Second Opinion**: Patients have the right to seek a second opinion from another healthcare provider, especially if they are unsure about a diagnosis or proposed treatment plan. Seeking a second opinion can provide peace of mind and additional insights.

●**The Right to Refuse Treatment**: You have the right to decline any treatment or procedure, even if it's recommended by your healthcare provider. Whether due to personal beliefs or concerns about the risks, you can make choices about your care.

●**The Right to Emergency Care**: In many countries, you are entitled to receive emergency care regardless of your ability to pay. Hospitals are required to provide stabilization and treatment for emergency conditions.

By being aware of these rights, you can advocate for yourself and ensure that you are treated with respect and fairness throughout your healthcare experience.

6.2 Obtaining Necessary Information

Engaging effectively with the healthcare system involves more than just visiting a doctor and receiving treatment. It's about actively participating in the process, ensuring that you understand your health situation, and acquiring the necessary information to make informed decisions. As we discussed earlier in this book, such as in Chapter 6.1 when exploring patient rights and specialist referrals, being proactive and well-prepared can make all the difference in navigating the complexities of healthcare. In this chapter, we focus on how to communicate with doctors, how to prepare for medical visits, and the key questions to ask during consultations to ensure that you leave your appointment feeling informed and confident.

How to Communicate with Doctors

Effective communication with your healthcare provider is the cornerstone of good medical care. When patients and doctors communicate well, it leads to better diagnoses, more tailored treatments, and a greater sense of partnership in managing health issues. However, this communication is often hampered by time constraints, medical jargon, and the overwhelming nature of some medical consultations.

As we have seen throughout this book, it is essential to be an active participant in your healthcare journey. Just as we've emphasized in other chapters the importance of monitoring health markers and taking ownership of lifestyle changes, engaging fully in conversations with your doctor is another step toward achieving better outcomes. Healthcare is a partnership, and communicating effectively with your doctor requires a thoughtful approach.

A critical aspect of doctor-patient communication is **clarity**. Many patients feel intimidated by medical jargon or may leave a consultation without fully understanding the diagnosis or treatment plan. This is a common issue but can be easily addressed. Doctors are trained professionals who should be able to explain complex health issues in simpler terms, and it's your right to ask for clarification. If your doctor uses a term or concept that you do not understand, don't hesitate to ask them to rephrase it in layman's terms. Clear communication not only helps you understand your situation but also ensures that you are more likely to follow through with treatment plans effectively.

In addition to understanding the language used, patients should feel empowered to ask about the reasoning behind diagnoses or suggested treatments. **Understanding the 'why'** behind a recommendation fosters confidence in the treatment process. If your doctor prescribes medication, for example, ask why that particular medication was chosen, what the expected outcomes are, and what potential side effects might occur. These conversations encourage shared decision-making, where you are not just a passive recipient of care but an active participant in choosing the best path forward.

Another key to effective communication is **providing accurate and complete information**. In Chapter 6.1, we touched on the importance of being honest with your healthcare provider about symptoms and medical history. This level of transparency is crucial for accurate diagnosis and treatment. Even minor symptoms or habits that might seem irrelevant can provide valuable insight into your overall health. For example, a seemingly unrelated issue such as sleep disturbances may be tied to larger conditions, such as stress or hormonal imbalances, and should not be overlooked. Being thorough in describing your symptoms and experiences helps your doctor get a clearer picture of your overall health and allows them to make better-informed decisions.

It's also important to express **any concerns or preferences** you may have regarding your care. If you have a preference for a particular type of treatment—whether it's a preference for non-pharmacological treatments or concerns about invasive procedures—communicate that openly. Healthcare should be a personalized experience, and your doctor should respect your values and preferences as they craft a care plan that suits you.

Furthermore, a productive relationship with your doctor depends on **trust**. Trust is built through open and respectful dialogue, where both patient and doctor understand that they are working toward a shared goal: your health and well-being. This trust is critical when you need to discuss sensitive topics, such as mental health concerns, lifestyle habits, or family history. These conversations may feel uncomfortable, but addressing them openly ensures that you receive the most comprehensive care possible.

Preparing for Medical Visits

Preparation is key to making the most out of your medical visits. As we discussed in Chapter 5.4, preparing for emergencies ensures you can respond effectively when health issues arise. Similarly, preparing for routine medical visits ensures that you make the best use of your doctor's time and leave the appointment with the information you need.

A well-prepared patient will have already thought about the key issues they want to address during the appointment. Before the visit, take time to reflect on your symptoms, questions, and concerns. Writing them down can be incredibly helpful, as it ensures that you don't forget to mention important details during the consultation. This can be particularly useful if you feel anxious or overwhelmed, as a prepared list helps keep the conversation focused and ensures that all your concerns are addressed.

Additionally, gather **relevant health information** before the visit. This includes a list of any medications you're currently taking, both prescription and over-the-counter, as well as supplements and vitamins. As we mentioned in Chapter 1 when discussing the importance of understanding biomarkers, keeping track of your current health metrics (such as weight, blood pressure, or cholesterol levels) can provide valuable context for your doctor. If you have seen other specialists or undergone recent tests, bring those results along to your appointment so that your doctor has the full picture.

It's also helpful to have a clear understanding of your **medical history**, including any previous illnesses, surgeries, or chronic conditions. This helps the doctor assess potential risk factors or patterns that may influence your current health. Moreover, if there is a family history of particular illnesses, such as heart disease or cancer, mention it to your doctor, as this can be relevant in determining your risk profile and guiding preventive measures.

In preparing for the visit, it's also important to **set expectations** for what you hope to achieve. Are you looking for a diagnosis? Do you need advice on managing an ongoing condition? Or are you simply looking for reassurance that your health is on track? Being clear about your goals for the appointment helps you and your doctor stay on the same page and ensures that the visit is productive.

Key Questions to Ask

Once you're in the consultation room, asking the right questions is essential to getting the information you need. Doctors may sometimes provide general explanations, so it's important to dig deeper into areas where you feel uncertain or where more details are required. As we've emphasized throughout this book, being an active participant in your health journey is crucial for achieving the best outcomes.

When discussing a **diagnosis**, it's important to ask your doctor for a clear explanation of the condition, including its causes, symptoms, and potential complications. Don't hesitate to ask, "What does this diagnosis mean for me?" Understanding the implications of a diagnosis allows you to take proactive steps in managing the condition.

It's helpful to ask how the condition might progress if left untreated and what lifestyle modifications could help improve your prognosis.

If your doctor recommends a **treatment plan**, ask about the pros and cons of the suggested approach. This includes understanding why a particular treatment was chosen, what the expected outcomes are, and what potential risks or side effects are involved. For example, if a medication is prescribed, inquire about how long it will take to see results, whether any interactions might occur with medications you're already taking, and what alternatives exist if you experience side effects.

Another important area of inquiry is **preventive care**. As discussed in Chapter 5.4, preventive strategies can greatly reduce the risk of illness. Ask your doctor about steps you can take to prevent the worsening of a condition or to avoid potential health risks altogether. Whether it's lifestyle changes, regular screenings, or vaccinations, preventive measures are an integral part of long-term health management.

When you feel uncertain about any aspect of your healthcare, don't hesitate to ask for a **second opinion**. As discussed in Chapter 6.1, patient rights include the ability to seek additional perspectives if you're unsure about a diagnosis or treatment plan. This is especially important for major decisions, such as surgery or long-term medication plans.

By preparing for your visits, communicating effectively, and asking the right questions, you can leave the doctor's office with confidence, knowing that you have the necessary information to make informed decisions about your health. In the end, healthcare is a partnership, and your active participation in the process is key to achieving the best possible outcomes.

6.3 Seeking Treatments and Therapies

Navigating the complex landscape of treatments and therapies can be one of the most challenging aspects of healthcare. Whether you're managing a chronic condition, recovering from an injury, or seeking preventive care, understanding the available treatment options and how to choose the right ones for your unique needs is critical to achieving the best outcomes. In this section, we will discuss the different types of treatments and therapies, the importance of integrative medicine, and the key factors to consider when choosing a treatment plan.

Available Treatment Options

When seeking medical care, it's essential to recognize that treatments vary widely depending on the condition being addressed, the patient's overall health, and the goals of care. Treatments generally fall into two main categories: **medical interventions** and **therapeutic approaches**. Both can be used together or separately, depending on the patient's needs, the severity of the condition, and the healthcare provider's recommendations.

Medical interventions include the use of medications, surgeries, or other procedural approaches to treat or manage diseases and conditions. These interventions are often based on standard medical practices and are guided by established research and clinical guidelines.

For example, if you are diagnosed with hypertension, your doctor might recommend medications such as ACE inhibitors or beta-blockers to manage your blood pressure. Similarly, in the case of heart disease, treatments might involve a combination of medication, lifestyle changes, and, in severe cases, surgical interventions like angioplasty or coronary artery bypass surgery. These types of treatments are commonly used for acute conditions or to manage chronic diseases that require ongoing attention.

Therapeutic approaches, on the other hand, focus more on rehabilitation, lifestyle adjustments, and holistic care. Physical therapy, occupational therapy, and psychological counseling fall into this category. For instance, after a knee surgery, physical therapy might be recommended to strengthen the surrounding muscles, improve mobility, and speed up recovery. Similarly, cognitive-behavioral therapy (CBT) is often used as part of mental health care to help patients manage anxiety, depression, or trauma.

In some cases, treatment plans will include a mix of both medical and therapeutic interventions. For example, someone recovering from a stroke may need medications to manage blood pressure and prevent future strokes while simultaneously undergoing physical therapy to regain mobility and speech therapy to recover communication skills.

The Importance of Integrative Medicine

As we have explored in earlier chapters, particularly in our discussion of holistic health in Chapter 5, maintaining overall health involves addressing both the body and the mind. This is where **integrative medicine** comes into play. Integrative medicine combines conventional Western medicine with alternative and complementary therapies, taking a holistic approach to patient care. It recognizes that treating a person means addressing more than just the symptoms of disease—it means taking into account their physical, emotional, mental, and even spiritual well-being.

For example, in managing chronic pain, an integrative approach might involve a combination of traditional pain medication, physical therapy, and complementary therapies such as acupuncture, massage therapy, or mindfulness meditation. These therapies are not intended to replace conventional medical treatments but rather to enhance their effectiveness by addressing other aspects of the patient's well-being.

Another key principle of integrative medicine is **patient-centered care**. This means that the treatment plan is tailored to the unique needs and preferences of the patient. In Chapter 6.1, we discussed the importance of choosing the right specialist and advocating for your healthcare preferences. Integrative medicine embraces this by allowing patients to be actively involved in their care decisions, ensuring that treatments align with their values and lifestyles.

For example, a cancer patient undergoing chemotherapy might choose to incorporate yoga, nutritional counseling, or stress-reduction techniques as part of their treatment plan to improve their quality of life during treatment. Integrative medicine recognizes that these complementary therapies can reduce side effects, enhance emotional well-being, and improve overall outcomes.

While integrative medicine is gaining recognition, it's essential to ensure that any complementary therapies are evidence-based and supported by clinical research. Working with a healthcare provider who understands both conventional and alternative treatments can help you navigate the options and make informed decisions about which therapies are appropriate for your condition.

Factors to Consider When Choosing Treatments

Choosing the right treatment plan is a highly individualized process and should be guided by several key factors. Understanding these factors will help you make informed decisions, ensuring that the chosen treatments align with your health goals and lifestyle while considering safety and efficacy.

One of the first things to consider is the **nature of your condition**. Acute conditions, such as infections or injuries, often require immediate, targeted interventions like antibiotics or surgery. Chronic conditions, such as diabetes or arthritis, often need long-term management strategies that include a combination of medication, lifestyle changes, and supportive therapies like physical therapy or dietary counseling.

For chronic conditions, it's important to think about **sustainability**. What treatments can you realistically maintain over the long term? For instance, if you have diabetes, managing your condition might involve taking medications, monitoring blood sugar, adhering to a specific diet, and exercising regularly. Choosing treatments that are sustainable and fit into your daily life is critical for maintaining your health over the long run.

Another important factor is **personal preferences and values**. As we discussed in Chapter 6.2, patient autonomy is a key aspect of navigating the healthcare system. When considering treatments, think about how they align with your preferences. Do you prefer non-invasive treatments when possible? Are you open to alternative therapies, or would you rather stick to conventional medical approaches? Communicating these preferences to your doctor can help ensure that your treatment plan reflects your values.

You should also consider the **side effects and risks** of any proposed treatment. Every medical intervention has potential risks, from minor side effects like nausea or headaches to more serious complications such as infections or blood clots. Weighing these risks against the potential benefits is crucial for making informed decisions. For example, if a medication has severe side effects, you may want to explore alternative options or adjust the dosage to minimize discomfort.

Another key consideration is **cost**. Treatments and therapies can vary widely in terms of expense, especially when factoring in insurance coverage, out-of-pocket costs, and the need for long-term management. For patients in countries without universal healthcare, navigating these costs can be especially challenging. In such cases, it's important to discuss the financial aspects of your treatment with your healthcare provider and explore options for cost-effective care, such as generic medications, alternative therapies covered by insurance, or community health programs.

For many patients, **quality of life** is an essential factor in choosing treatments. Some treatments may be highly effective at managing or curing a condition but can significantly reduce your quality of life, whether due to side effects, recovery time, or lifestyle restrictions. When evaluating treatment options, consider how each will impact your ability to live a fulfilling, active life. For example, aggressive chemotherapy might be the most effective treatment for cancer, but if it significantly reduces quality of life, some patients may opt for palliative care or other less invasive treatments that prioritize comfort.

Finally, it's essential to remember that choosing a treatment is not always a **one-time decision**. Healthcare is a dynamic process, and as your condition changes or as new treatments become available, your treatment plan may need to be adjusted. As we explored in Chapter 5 when discussing resilience, adapting to change is a key part of managing health. Regularly reviewing and reassessing your treatment plan with your healthcare provider ensures that it continues to meet your needs and goals over time.

The Importance of Collaborative Decision-Making

Choosing a treatment plan should always be a **collaborative process** between you and your healthcare provider. As we have emphasized throughout this book, patient autonomy is critical in making healthcare decisions. Shared decision-making means that your doctor provides expert guidance, but you remain an active participant in the final choice.

During this process, don't be afraid to **ask questions**. In Chapter 6.2, we discussed the importance of clear communication with your doctor, and this remains essential when discussing treatment options. If you don't understand why a specific treatment is being recommended, ask your doctor to explain the reasoning behind it. If you have concerns about side effects or risks, express them openly. You have the right to fully understand every aspect of your care before making a decision.

If you're unsure about a recommended treatment, seeking a **second opinion** is also a valuable option. As mentioned in Chapter 6.1, obtaining a second opinion can provide new insights or confirm the initial recommendation, giving you greater confidence in your treatment choice. It's especially important to consider a second opinion for serious conditions, such as cancer or heart disease, where multiple treatment options may be available, each with different risks and benefits.

Ultimately, the goal of treatment is not just to manage or cure a condition but to help you achieve the best possible quality of life. By understanding the available options, weighing the risks and benefits, and working collaboratively with your healthcare provider, you can create a treatment plan that supports your health and well-being in the long term.

6.4 Self-Management of Health

Taking an active role in managing your health is one of the most empowering steps you can take toward long-term well-being. As we've discussed throughout this book, particularly in earlier sections on nutrition, exercise, and resilience, personal health isn't just something that happens to you—it's something you can control, influence, and improve through conscious actions. In this chapter, we'll explore how to become a proactive patient, track symptoms and progress, and use self-help resources to stay on top of your health and prevent potential problems before they arise.

How to Become a Proactive Patient

Being a proactive patient means taking charge of your health in a way that ensures you receive the best possible care. It's about more than just going to appointments when you feel unwell; it's about staying informed, being prepared, and engaging with your healthcare providers as an active participant in your care.

One of the first steps toward becoming a proactive patient is to **educate yourself** about your health conditions or any risk factors that may impact your well-being. Knowledge is power, and the more you understand about your body and how it works, the better equipped you will be to make informed decisions about your care. As we've seen in earlier chapters, such as Chapter 6.2 on obtaining necessary information, understanding the reasoning behind medical advice can make a significant difference in how well you follow through with treatment plans. Don't hesitate to ask your doctor detailed questions, and consider researching reputable sources like government health websites, medical journals, and books to deepen your understanding.

Another important aspect of being a proactive patient is **taking responsibility for your lifestyle choices**. Many chronic conditions, such as heart disease, diabetes, and hypertension, are directly influenced by factors like diet, exercise, and stress management. In Chapter 2, we discussed the importance of a balanced diet, and in Chapter 4, we covered the health benefits of regular physical activity. These lifestyle choices are not just recommendations—they are critical components of self-management that can dramatically improve your quality of life and reduce the need for medical interventions down the road.

Being proactive also means **building a strong relationship with your healthcare providers**. As we discussed in Chapter 6.3, shared decision-making is essential for effective care. To foster this relationship, it's important to maintain open communication with your doctors and nurses, actively participate in discussions about your treatment, and keep them informed about any changes in your health. If you feel that something isn't working or you have concerns about side effects, don't hesitate to voice those concerns. Being honest and transparent with your doctor allows them to adjust your care plan to better suit your needs.

Proactive patients are also **organized**. Keep track of your medical history, including past diagnoses, treatments, and any medications you are currently taking. This not only makes it easier for your healthcare provider to give you appropriate care, but it also allows you to have a clear understanding of your health over time. Maintain an updated list of any allergies, surgeries, and chronic conditions so you can provide accurate information when needed. In Chapter 6.1, we touched on the importance of keeping this information readily available, especially when seeing specialists or new healthcare providers.

Finally, being a proactive patient means **being vigilant about preventive care**. Don't wait for symptoms to appear before you seek medical attention. As discussed in Chapter 5.4, preventive strategies like vaccinations, regular screenings, and health checkups are essential for catching problems early and avoiding more serious conditions. Schedule routine exams, blood tests, and cancer screenings according to your age, gender, and family history, and make sure you stay up-to-date with your immunizations.

Tracking Symptoms and Progress

An important part of self-managing your health is keeping track of your symptoms and any progress you make with treatment or lifestyle changes. Monitoring your health over time not only helps you detect patterns and identify potential issues early but also provides your doctor with valuable data that can inform their decisions about your care.

Symptom tracking is especially useful for chronic conditions like asthma, diabetes, migraines, or arthritis, where symptoms can fluctuate based on triggers, medications, or changes in routine. By keeping a detailed record of your symptoms, including their frequency, intensity, and any accompanying factors, you can help your doctor get a clearer picture of what might be contributing to flare-ups or exacerbations. For example, if you suffer from migraines, tracking when they occur, what you were doing beforehand, and any foods you ate can help identify potential triggers and lead to better treatment.

Similarly, **tracking your progress** with treatments and lifestyle changes helps you assess what is working and what needs adjustment. If your doctor prescribes a new medication, it's important to note how you feel after starting it, whether it alleviates your symptoms, and if you experience any side effects. If you're implementing lifestyle changes—such as a new exercise routine or dietary adjustments—tracking how these changes affect your energy levels, mood, or physical health can help you stay motivated and identify areas for improvement.

There are several ways to track symptoms and progress:

1. **Journaling**: A simple way to start tracking your health is by keeping a daily or weekly journal. You can jot down your symptoms, medications, diet, exercise, and any other factors that might influence your health. This not only serves as a record for your doctor but also helps you become more in tune with your body.

2. **Mobile apps**: Today, there are numerous health-tracking apps available that make it easy to log symptoms, track your progress, and share this information with your healthcare provider. Apps like **MyFitnessPal**, **Headspace**, or condition-specific apps like **Migraine Buddy** offer an easy way to monitor health metrics over time. These apps can also provide reminders for medications, appointments, and other aspects of your care.

3. **Wearable devices**: Fitness trackers and smartwatches can also play a role in self-management by monitoring things like heart rate, sleep patterns, physical activity, and

calorie intake. These devices provide real-time data that you can share with your doctor, helping them assess your overall health more accurately.

Regardless of how you track your symptoms and progress, the key is **consistency**. Keeping detailed records over time allows you and your doctor to make more informed decisions about your care. It also helps you take control of your health by offering a clear picture of how your body responds to various treatments and lifestyle changes.

Self-Help Resources

Self-management doesn't end with tracking symptoms and maintaining communication with your healthcare provider. Many **self-help resources** are available to help you stay informed, adopt healthier habits, and manage your well-being more effectively.

First and foremost, **online health portals** offered by many healthcare providers allow you to access your medical records, view test results, schedule appointments, and even communicate with your doctor online. These tools give you direct access to important health information and allow you to take care of many aspects of your health without needing to make frequent in-person visits.

In addition to online portals, **educational websites** provide valuable information about specific health conditions, treatments, and preventive measures. Websites like **MedlinePlus**, the **Mayo Clinic**, and the **Centers for Disease Control and Prevention (CDC)** offer reliable, evidence-based information that can help you understand your condition and make informed decisions about your care. As mentioned in Chapter 6.3, it's important to use reputable sources to avoid misinformation, especially when researching health topics online.

Support groups are another valuable resource for self-management. Whether you're managing a chronic condition or going through a difficult period in your life, connecting with others who share similar experiences can provide emotional support, practical advice, and a sense of community. In Chapter 5.5, we discussed the importance of a supportive community, and support groups—whether in person or online—can play a critical role in maintaining mental and emotional health. Many hospitals and health organizations offer support groups for specific conditions like cancer, diabetes, or mental health disorders, and online forums such as those found on **Reddit** or **Facebook** provide additional spaces for people to share experiences and offer support.

For those looking to adopt healthier habits, **wellness programs** and **self-help books** can be powerful tools. Many workplaces offer wellness programs that provide access to fitness resources, stress management tools, and nutritional counseling. Self-help books on topics such as stress reduction, fitness, and mental health can also offer valuable guidance for implementing positive lifestyle changes.

Lastly, consider seeking out **professional resources**, such as health coaches, nutritionists, or therapists, who can offer personalized guidance and help you stay accountable to your health goals. These professionals can provide tailored advice, help you navigate challenges, and work with you to develop a sustainable plan for long-term health.

By combining proactive care, symptom tracking, and the use of self-help resources, you can take control of your health journey and stay on top of any challenges that arise. Self-management isn't about replacing professional healthcare—it's about complementing it with informed, empowered decision-making and a consistent commitment to your own well-being.

6.5 Advocating for Your Health

Taking control of your health journey extends beyond just self-management and tracking symptoms. It involves actively advocating for your needs, making informed decisions, and ensuring that you receive the best possible care. Advocacy is a critical aspect of being an empowered patient, as it helps ensure your voice is heard in a healthcare system that can sometimes feel overwhelming or impersonal. In this chapter, we will explore how to advocate for your health, how to stand up for your rights, the role of public health initiatives, and why health awareness is crucial to making informed decisions.

How to Stand Up for Your Rights

Being a proactive patient also means standing up for your rights in the healthcare system. As we discussed in Chapter 6.1, knowing your patient rights is a fundamental part of navigating the system. Healthcare providers are obligated to provide respectful, fair, and unbiased care, but it is also important for patients to be aware of their own power in the relationship. You have the right to ask questions, seek clarification, and voice concerns when necessary.

One of the most important aspects of advocating for your rights is **assertive communication**. This means clearly and confidently expressing your needs, preferences, and concerns during medical consultations. For example, if a treatment plan doesn't feel right to you, or if you have concerns about side effects, speak up. Your doctor should listen to you, and if they don't, you may want to consider seeking care from another provider who respects your input. Remember, healthcare is a partnership, and your participation is crucial to its success.

It's equally important to ask for **second opinions** if you feel uncertain about a diagnosis or treatment plan. As we explored in Chapter 6.3, seeking a second opinion is a standard practice, especially for major health decisions like surgeries or long-term treatments. By consulting another expert, you gain different perspectives, which can either confirm your current plan or offer new options that you hadn't considered. Don't hesitate to advocate for this right, particularly when it comes to significant decisions regarding your health.

Another key right is the ability to **access your medical records**. Under privacy laws like HIPAA (Health Insurance Portability and Accountability Act) in the United States, you have the right to view and request copies of your health information. This includes lab results, imaging reports, doctors' notes, and any other relevant documentation about your care. Keeping copies of your medical records allows you to stay informed about your health and ensures that you have the information you need when seeing multiple providers.

Additionally, standing up for your rights means **knowing when to challenge medical advice**. While healthcare professionals have the expertise and experience to provide recommendations, you are the ultimate decision-maker in your health care. If a treatment feels overly aggressive, unnecessary, or conflicts with your personal values, it's important to voice those concerns. This isn't about rejecting professional advice, but rather ensuring that the care you receive aligns with your preferences and goals. For instance, some patients might prefer to avoid certain medications or surgical procedures in favor of alternative treatments or more conservative approaches. Being clear about these preferences helps guide your healthcare team to craft a treatment plan that suits you.

Involvement in Public Health Initiatives

Beyond advocating for your own individual care, another powerful way to influence health outcomes is through involvement in **public health initiatives**. Public health campaigns, policies, and programs are designed to promote well-being at a societal level, focusing on prevention, education, and access to care. By participating in these initiatives, you not only contribute to your own health but also support broader community efforts to improve healthcare for everyone.

One way to get involved is by **supporting preventive health campaigns**, such as those that promote vaccination, cancer screenings, or healthy living. These initiatives often rely on public engagement to spread awareness and encourage participation in preventive measures. For instance, campaigns that focus on flu vaccination can significantly reduce the spread of illness in communities, particularly among vulnerable populations. By participating in these programs, whether through advocating for vaccination or spreading awareness on social media, you contribute to the greater good of public health.

Another area of involvement is **advocating for health equity**. Health equity initiatives aim to reduce disparities in healthcare access and outcomes across different populations, particularly those affected by socioeconomic, racial, or geographic barriers. Advocacy efforts may focus on increasing access to healthcare services in underserved areas, improving maternal care for minority women, or supporting mental health services in rural communities. By raising awareness, supporting policies that address these disparities, and volunteering with organizations that work on these issues, you become part of a broader movement to make healthcare more inclusive and accessible.

For those who are passionate about healthcare reform, **advocating for policy changes** can be an effective way to promote systemic improvements. Healthcare policy affects everything from insurance coverage and drug pricing to access to services and public health funding. Engaging with policymakers, participating in public hearings, or joining health advocacy groups allows individuals to influence the policies that shape the healthcare system. For example, advocacy for expanded access to telemedicine has grown in recent years, driven by the need for remote care during the COVID-19 pandemic. By supporting these efforts, you can help create a more adaptable and accessible healthcare system for all.

The Importance of Health Awareness

At the heart of effective health advocacy is **awareness**. Being aware of your own health status, as well as current health trends and recommendations, allows you to make informed choices and advocate for better care. This awareness begins with understanding your body and recognizing changes that could signal potential health problems, as we discussed in Chapter 6.4 on self-management.

In addition to self-awareness, staying up-to-date on **medical research and guidelines** is essential for informed advocacy. Healthcare is a rapidly evolving field, with new treatments, technologies, and evidence-based practices emerging regularly. By keeping informed about the latest developments, you can engage more confidently with your healthcare providers and ask pertinent questions. For example, if new research suggests a more effective treatment for your condition, you can discuss it with your doctor to see if it's appropriate for your care. Subscribing to reputable health newsletters, reading medical journals, and attending health seminars or workshops can help you stay informed.

Health literacy is another crucial aspect of awareness. Health literacy refers to the ability to understand health information and use it to make appropriate decisions. Low health literacy can lead to misunderstandings about treatment options, medication usage, and preventive care, which can negatively impact health outcomes. To improve health literacy, take time to ask questions during medical appointments, read educational materials from reliable sources, and seek clarification on anything that seems unclear. The more you understand about your health, the better equipped you will be to advocate for yourself effectively.

Public awareness campaigns also play a critical role in promoting health literacy on a broader scale. From educating people about the dangers of smoking to promoting the benefits of regular exercise and balanced diets, these campaigns provide the knowledge people need to take control of their health. Engaging with these campaigns, whether through social media, community outreach, or educational events, helps spread important health messages that benefit society as a whole.

In addition to raising awareness about specific health issues, these campaigns often encourage **early detection and intervention**, which are key to preventing more serious health problems. For instance, awareness campaigns for breast cancer encourage women to schedule mammograms, while campaigns for heart disease promote regular blood pressure checks and cholesterol monitoring. By staying informed and encouraging others to participate in preventive care, you contribute to a culture of proactive health management.

Advocating for your health is about taking an active role in both your personal healthcare and in the broader public health landscape. From standing up for your rights during medical appointments to participating in public health initiatives, advocacy is an essential component of managing your well-being. As we've seen throughout this book, self-management, education, and proactive communication with healthcare providers are key factors in achieving the best possible outcomes. By combining these efforts with broader advocacy for health equity and preventive care, you contribute to a healthcare system that benefits not only yourself but also your community.

Ultimately, health advocacy empowers you to be in control of your healthcare decisions, ensuring that you receive the best care tailored to your needs while also contributing to the larger goal of improving health outcomes for everyone.

Chapter 7: Environmental Factors and Metabolism

Our environment plays a significant role in shaping our metabolic health. From the air we breathe to the toxins we are exposed to daily, these environmental factors can either support or disrupt the body's delicate metabolic balance. As more research uncovers the profound effects of our surroundings on health, it becomes clear that optimizing our environment is crucial for metabolic wellness.

Environmental factors such as pollution, exposure to toxins, and even electromagnetic fields (EMFs) can contribute to inflammation, oxidative stress, and metabolic dysfunction. Meanwhile, positive environmental exposures—like sunlight, clean air, and balanced temperatures—can enhance mitochondrial function, improve cellular health, and support overall metabolism.

In this chapter, we will delve into how environmental toxins, air quality, sunlight exposure, and other external factors impact metabolic health. We will explore strategies to reduce exposure to harmful environmental influences and introduce simple lifestyle adaptations that can help your body thrive in a world filled with potential environmental stressors.

7.1 How Environmental Toxins Affect Cellular Health

The environment we live in has a profound impact on our metabolic health. Our cells are the engines of our body, and just like any engine, they rely on clean, efficient fuel to function optimally. However, in today's world, we are constantly exposed to a wide range of environmental toxins that can hinder cellular function and disrupt metabolism. These toxins come from various sources—air pollution, contaminated water, pesticides, plastics, and even household cleaning products. While some exposure is inevitable, understanding how these toxins affect our bodies and taking steps to minimize them is crucial for maintaining good metabolic health.

The first challenge we face is that many of these toxins are **invisible** to us in our daily lives, making it easy to overlook their impact. For example, heavy metals such as lead, mercury, and cadmium can accumulate in the body over time, causing oxidative stress. This stress damages our cells' ability to generate energy efficiently, leading to fatigue, weakened immune function, and even chronic disease. Another common group of toxins, called endocrine disruptors, interfere with our hormonal balance, which—as we saw in Chapter 9—is critical for regulating metabolism. Chemicals like bisphenol A (BPA), commonly found in plastics, can mimic hormones in the body and lead to weight gain, insulin resistance, and other metabolic disorders.

These **disruptions at the cellular level** often go unnoticed until they manifest as symptoms. A slow, underlying accumulation of toxins can lead to chronic inflammation, a condition closely linked to metabolic dysfunction. Inflammation is our body's natural response to harmful stimuli, but when it's triggered constantly by environmental toxins, it becomes chronic and contributes to conditions such as heart disease, diabetes, and obesity. As we've discussed earlier in the book, addressing the root causes of inflammation is essential for restoring metabolic balance and preventing disease.

In addition to toxins affecting our body's natural ability to produce energy, they also interfere with the **detoxification process** itself. Our liver, kidneys, and skin are all part of the detoxification system, designed to neutralize and eliminate harmful substances. But when the body is overwhelmed with too many toxins, these organs can become overworked, reducing their efficiency. The liver, for example, is responsible for filtering toxins from the blood and converting them into less harmful substances that can be safely excreted. If the liver is overburdened, it becomes less effective at breaking down fats, processing nutrients, and regulating blood sugar—key functions that are directly linked to metabolic health.

To support our detoxification system, it's essential to focus on reducing exposure to **common environmental toxins**. This doesn't mean we can eliminate every single harmful chemical from our lives, but there are practical steps we can take to reduce the burden. Start by evaluating the products you use daily, such as household cleaners, cosmetics, and plastic containers. Many of these products contain chemicals like phthalates, parabens, and volatile organic compounds (VOCs) that contribute to metabolic imbalance. Switching to natural, non-toxic alternatives can reduce the number of harmful chemicals your body needs to process.

Another effective strategy is to **focus on improving air and water quality**. Indoor air pollution is often worse than outdoor air, especially when we're exposed to off-gassing from furniture, paints, and cleaning products. Installing air purifiers, using natural cleaning products, and ventilating your home regularly can help minimize these pollutants. Similarly, ensuring that your drinking water is free from contaminants like lead, chlorine, and pesticides is crucial. Investing in a high-quality water filtration system is one of the simplest ways to ensure your body isn't burdened by toxins from this vital source.

Our diet plays a critical role in how well we handle environmental toxins. Foods rich in **antioxidants**—such as berries, leafy greens, and nuts—help neutralize the oxidative stress caused by toxins. These foods are not just supportive in detoxifying harmful chemicals; they also protect cells from further damage. Fiber is another key nutrient in supporting the body's detox processes. It binds to toxins in the digestive tract, helping to flush them out through bowel movements, preventing reabsorption into the bloodstream.

Moreover, as we learned in Chapter 5, practices like **heat exposure** through saunas can also play a role in detoxification. Sweating is one of the body's natural ways of eliminating toxins. Regular sauna use has been shown to enhance the removal of heavy metals and other toxins through the skin, providing another layer of support to the liver and kidneys.

When it comes to detoxification, one of the most overlooked factors is **hydration**. Water is essential for flushing toxins out of the body through urine and sweat. Dehydration slows down this process, allowing toxins to accumulate in the body. Ensuring proper hydration is a simple yet powerful tool for improving detoxification efficiency, allowing the liver and kidneys to function optimally.

It's important to remember that detoxification is not about extreme cleanses or deprivation diets, which can often do more harm than good. Instead, think of it as an ongoing, **gentle support system** for your body's natural processes. By minimizing exposure to harmful chemicals and providing your body with the right nutrients, hydration, and lifestyle habits, you can reduce the toxic burden on your system and improve your metabolic function. The key to thriving in a world filled with environmental toxins is not through avoidance but through balance and making small, sustainable changes.

As we continue to explore other aspects of resilience and metabolic health, it's clear that detoxification and environmental awareness form a foundation for overall well-being. Our cells, like any machine, perform better when they're running clean and fueled with the right nutrients. By understanding how toxins impact cellular health, we empower ourselves to make choices that support optimal metabolism and long-term vitality.

7.2 Building Resilience Through Cold and Heat Exposure

Our bodies have evolved over millennia to adapt to a wide range of environmental stressors, from extreme cold to intense heat. This ability to endure and thrive in varying conditions is a testament to human resilience. Today, in an age where climate-controlled environments are the norm, we often lose touch with the natural extremes that once shaped our survival. However, cold and heat exposure can still play a vital role in optimizing our health, especially when it comes to metabolic function. These environmental stressors trigger adaptive responses in the body that promote cellular efficiency, enhance energy production, and ultimately improve overall metabolic health.

Metabolic Benefits of Cold Therapy

Cold exposure is not a new concept, though it has gained popularity in recent years through practices like cold showers, ice baths, and cryotherapy. Historically, cold water immersion has been used in various cultures to stimulate recovery, improve circulation, and boost physical resilience. From a metabolic perspective, cold therapy has a unique ability to activate **brown adipose tissue (BAT)**, commonly referred to as brown fat. Unlike white fat, which stores energy, brown fat burns calories to generate heat in a process known as **non-shivering thermogenesis**.

This process is crucial for maintaining body temperature when exposed to cold environments, but it also has profound effects on metabolic health. When brown fat is activated, it burns glucose and fat to produce heat, which not only helps to increase overall energy expenditure but also improves glucose metabolism. Individuals with higher levels of active brown fat tend to have better insulin sensitivity and are at a lower risk of developing metabolic disorders such as type 2 diabetes. As we explored in Chapter 9, maintaining optimal insulin sensitivity is essential for metabolic health, and cold therapy offers a natural way to enhance this process.

Cold exposure also promotes the release of **norepinephrine**, a hormone and neurotransmitter that plays a key role in regulating metabolism, focus, and mood. When the body is exposed to cold, norepinephrine levels increase, which has anti-inflammatory effects and helps improve metabolic efficiency. Inflammation, as we've discussed earlier in the book, is a major contributor to metabolic dysfunction. By reducing chronic inflammation, cold therapy supports healthier cellular function and promotes an overall metabolic balance. In addition to its anti-inflammatory properties, norepinephrine helps break down fat stores, making cold exposure a useful tool for those seeking to improve fat metabolism and body composition.

Another significant benefit of cold therapy is its impact on the **mitochondria**, the energy powerhouses of our cells. Cold exposure stimulates mitochondrial biogenesis, which is the process by which new mitochondria are formed within cells. This enhances the body's ability to produce energy more efficiently, which translates into better endurance, improved recovery, and increased resilience to physical stress. As we saw in Chapter 4, efficient energy production is critical for maintaining physical activity levels, and cold exposure can support this by optimizing mitochondrial function.

Incorporating cold therapy into your routine doesn't require extreme measures. It can begin with something as simple as ending your daily shower with 30 seconds of cold water. This brief exposure is enough to trigger the body's adaptive responses without overwhelming your system. Over time, as your tolerance builds, you can extend the duration or explore more intense methods, such as ice baths or outdoor cold immersion. For those interested in exploring the full benefits of cold therapy, regular cryotherapy sessions—where the body is briefly exposed to temperatures as low as -200°F—can offer a more controlled environment to experience the metabolic advantages of extreme cold.

Heat Exposure and Its Impact on Cellular Function

While cold exposure promotes metabolic activity through brown fat activation and mitochondrial biogenesis, heat therapy works in a different but equally powerful way to improve metabolic health. The practice of using heat for therapeutic purposes has been part of many cultures for centuries. Saunas, steam rooms, and hot springs have long been valued for their healing properties, particularly in promoting detoxification and relaxation.

Today, science is uncovering how these traditional practices support metabolic function at the cellular level.

One of the primary benefits of heat exposure is the **activation of heat shock proteins (HSPs)**. These proteins play a crucial role in protecting cells from stress, promoting the repair of damaged proteins, and maintaining cellular homeostasis. When the body is exposed to heat, HSPs help to stabilize and refold damaged proteins that may have become misfolded due to stress, aging, or disease. This cellular repair process not only enhances metabolic efficiency but also supports longevity by ensuring that cells function optimally for as long as possible.

Heat exposure also stimulates the production of **growth hormone**, a key regulator of metabolism, muscle repair, and fat burning. As we age, our natural levels of growth hormone decline, contributing to the gradual slowdown of metabolism and the loss of muscle mass. Regular heat exposure, such as through sauna use, has been shown to increase growth hormone production, which can help counteract these age-related metabolic changes. By promoting muscle repair and enhancing fat metabolism, heat therapy supports the maintenance of a lean body composition and optimal metabolic health, even in later life.

Another critical way in which heat exposure impacts metabolic function is through its effect on the **cardiovascular system**. When the body is exposed to heat, blood vessels dilate, and heart rate increases, mimicking the effects of moderate exercise. This increase in circulation delivers more oxygen and nutrients to cells, promoting better energy production and metabolic efficiency. Improved circulation also supports the removal of metabolic waste products, which helps prevent the buildup of toxins that can impair cellular function. As we explored in Chapter 7.1, detoxification is essential for maintaining a healthy metabolism, and heat therapy enhances this process by encouraging thermoregulatory sweating. Through sweating, the body can eliminate harmful substances like heavy metals, bisphenol A (BPA), and other environmental toxins that can disrupt metabolic processes.

In addition to its physical benefits, heat exposure has a positive effect on **mental health**, which, as we discussed in Chapter 8, is closely linked to metabolic well-being. The deep relaxation that comes from spending time in a sauna or steam room can reduce stress, lower cortisol levels, and improve mood. Since chronic stress and elevated cortisol levels are major contributors to metabolic disorders, reducing stress through heat exposure supports a more balanced metabolism. Furthermore, the meditative quality of heat therapy—whether it's in the form of a sauna session or hot yoga—can help cultivate mindfulness, which has been shown to improve both mental and metabolic health.

For those new to heat therapy, it's important to approach it gradually. Starting with shorter sauna sessions of 10-15 minutes can help your body acclimate to the heat. Over time, you can increase the duration to 20-30 minutes, ensuring that you stay hydrated throughout the process. Hydration is crucial when practicing heat therapy, as the body loses water and electrolytes through sweating. Replenishing these fluids is essential for maintaining metabolic function and preventing dehydration, which can impair energy production.

Incorporating heat therapy into your lifestyle can be as simple as using a sauna or steam room once or twice a week. For individuals who prefer more physical engagement, hot yoga offers a combination of heat exposure and physical activity, both of which contribute to improved metabolic health. Regardless of the method you choose, regular heat exposure is a powerful way to enhance resilience, support cellular function, and maintain a healthy metabolism.

By engaging with both cold and heat exposure, the body builds a balanced and adaptable metabolic system capable of thriving in various conditions. As we have seen throughout the book, achieving metabolic health is not just about internal factors like diet and exercise; it's also about how we interact with our external environment. Cold and heat exposure provide natural, accessible methods to optimize energy production, reduce inflammation, and support long-term health.

7.3 Air Quality and Its Impact on Health

The quality of the air we breathe is often an overlooked component of health, yet it plays a significant role in both metabolic and respiratory functions. While much attention is given to nutrition, exercise, and sleep, the air we inhale daily can have a profound influence on our cellular health and overall metabolic efficiency. Poor air quality, particularly due to pollution, can contribute to systemic inflammation, oxidative stress, and metabolic dysfunction, which in turn affect energy production, immune function, and respiratory health. As we examine the intricate ways the environment shapes metabolic health, it's essential to understand the consequences of breathing polluted air and the steps we can take to mitigate its impact.

The Effects of Pollution on Metabolic and Respiratory Health

Air pollution has become a growing concern in many parts of the world, with urban areas and industrial regions being particularly affected. Pollutants such as particulate matter (PM), nitrogen dioxide (NO2), sulfur dioxide (SO2), and volatile organic compounds (VOCs) are common in outdoor air, and they can easily penetrate indoor environments as well. These pollutants, especially fine particulate matter (PM2.5), are small enough to be inhaled deep into the lungs, where they can enter the bloodstream and spread throughout the body. Once in the bloodstream, these particles can cause widespread inflammation and oxidative stress, disrupting both metabolic and respiratory systems.

One of the most immediate impacts of poor air quality is on respiratory health. Inhaling polluted air can irritate the airways, leading to chronic respiratory conditions like asthma, chronic obstructive pulmonary disease (COPD), and bronchitis. These conditions not only affect breathing but also strain the cardiovascular system, as the body struggles to deliver adequate oxygen to tissues. Over time, this can lead to reduced oxygen supply to cells, impairing their ability to produce energy efficiently. As we've discussed in earlier chapters, cellular energy production is at the core of metabolic health, and anything that hampers this process can have long-term consequences for overall well-being.

The inflammatory response triggered by air pollution is not limited to the lungs; it affects the entire body. Inflammation is a natural defense mechanism designed to protect the body from harmful substances, but when it becomes chronic, it can lead to metabolic disturbances. Exposure to pollutants has been linked to insulin resistance, a condition where cells become less responsive to insulin, making it harder for the body to regulate blood sugar levels. This contributes to the development of metabolic disorders such as type 2 diabetes and obesity. As we explored in Chapter 9, insulin resistance is a major risk factor for many chronic diseases, and poor air quality can exacerbate this issue by promoting systemic inflammation.

Pollution also plays a role in the development of **oxidative stress**, a condition where there is an imbalance between free radicals and antioxidants in the body. Free radicals are unstable molecules that can damage cells, proteins, and DNA, leading to premature aging and the onset of diseases. When pollution enters the body, it increases the production of free radicals, overwhelming the body's natural antioxidant defenses. This oxidative damage can impair mitochondrial function—the energy powerhouses of our cells—resulting in reduced energy production and increased fatigue. Over time, this can lead to a decline in metabolic function, making it harder for the body to maintain a healthy weight, regulate blood sugar, and recover from physical activity.

Another key way in which air pollution impacts metabolic health is through its effect on the **gut microbiome**. Recent studies have shown that inhaled pollutants can alter the composition of gut bacteria, leading to dysbiosis, a condition where the balance of healthy and harmful bacteria in the gut is disrupted. As we discussed in Chapter 8, the gut microbiome plays a critical role in metabolic health, influencing everything from digestion to immune function. By disrupting the gut microbiome, air pollution can contribute to metabolic imbalances, increasing the risk of conditions like obesity, diabetes, and cardiovascular disease.

Strategies to Improve Indoor Air Quality

While we may have little control over outdoor air quality, there are several strategies we can implement to improve the air we breathe indoors. Given that most people spend a significant portion of their day inside—whether at home, at work, or in other indoor environments—it's crucial to focus on reducing exposure to indoor pollutants. Indoor air quality is often compromised by sources such as cleaning products, furniture, carpets, and building materials, all of which can release VOCs and other harmful chemicals into the air. Additionally, dust, pet dander, mold, and tobacco smoke can further degrade the air quality in enclosed spaces.

One of the most effective ways to improve indoor air quality is through **ventilation**. Proper ventilation allows fresh air to circulate throughout the space, diluting indoor pollutants and removing stale air. Opening windows and doors regularly, especially in well-insulated homes, can help maintain good air circulation. For those living in areas where outdoor pollution is a concern, it may be beneficial to use mechanical ventilation systems with air filters that can remove particulate matter and other pollutants from the incoming air.

Another valuable tool for improving air quality is the use of **air purifiers**. These devices are designed to filter out airborne particles, allergens, and pollutants, making the indoor environment cleaner and safer to breathe. When choosing an air purifier, it's important to look for one that has a **high-efficiency particulate air (HEPA) filter**, as this type of filter is capable of capturing even the smallest particles, such as PM2.5, which can penetrate deep into the lungs and enter the bloodstream. HEPA filters can be particularly helpful for individuals with respiratory conditions or allergies, as they remove allergens like dust, pollen, and pet dander, reducing the risk of irritation and inflammation.

Reducing the use of **toxic cleaning products** and **synthetic air fresheners** is another crucial step in improving indoor air quality. Many household cleaning products contain VOCs that can linger in the air long after they've been used, contributing to indoor air pollution. Switching to natural, non-toxic cleaning products made from ingredients like vinegar, baking soda, and essential oils can significantly reduce your exposure to these harmful chemicals. Similarly, avoiding synthetic air fresheners and scented candles, which often contain phthalates and other chemicals, can help minimize indoor pollution. Instead, opt for natural air fresheners, such as essential oil diffusers or simply opening windows to let fresh air in.

Houseplants can also play a role in improving air quality. While their impact may be limited compared to mechanical filtration, certain plants, such as spider plants, snake plants, and peace lilies, have been shown to remove small amounts of VOCs and carbon dioxide from the air. In addition to their aesthetic and mental health benefits, houseplants can contribute to a healthier indoor environment by naturally purifying the air.

Finally, maintaining clean indoor spaces is essential for minimizing exposure to dust, mold, and other allergens that can negatively affect both respiratory and metabolic health. Regularly cleaning surfaces, vacuuming carpets with a HEPA filter vacuum, and controlling humidity levels (between 30-50%) can help prevent the growth of mold and reduce dust accumulation. Mold, in particular, can be a serious issue for both metabolic and respiratory health, as it releases spores that can trigger inflammation and allergic reactions.

Long-Term Benefits of Clean Air on Metabolism

Breathing clean air has far-reaching benefits for both metabolic and respiratory health, extending well beyond the immediate effects on the lungs. By reducing exposure to pollutants, the body can maintain better oxygen delivery to cells, enhancing cellular respiration and energy production. Over time, this leads to improved stamina, reduced fatigue, and more efficient metabolic function. With less systemic inflammation and oxidative stress, the body is better equipped to regulate blood sugar, manage weight, and support cardiovascular health.

As we've discussed in previous chapters, chronic inflammation is a key driver of metabolic disorders, and reducing exposure to environmental pollutants is one of the most effective ways to lower inflammation levels. Clean air also supports better hormonal balance, as pollution-related inflammation can disrupt hormone signaling, contributing to insulin resistance and weight gain. By improving air quality, you create an environment where your cells can thrive, ultimately enhancing metabolic resilience and reducing the risk of developing chronic diseases.

Furthermore, maintaining good air quality can have a positive impact on **mental clarity** and **cognitive function**, both of which are closely linked to metabolic health. Breathing clean air helps reduce oxidative stress in the brain, supporting better focus, memory, and decision-making abilities. As we explored in Chapter 8, mental health is deeply connected to metabolic well-being, and optimizing air quality is one more way to support both.

Air quality is a critical but often overlooked factor in metabolic health. By understanding how pollution affects both respiratory and metabolic systems, and by taking proactive steps to improve the air we breathe, we can reduce inflammation, support cellular function, and enhance overall well-being.

7.4 The Role of Sunlight and Vitamin D

Sunlight is one of the most powerful and natural influences on human health, and its importance extends far beyond its role in vision or warmth. Regular sunlight exposure is essential for optimizing metabolic health, influencing everything from mitochondrial function to hormonal balance. One of the most critical benefits of sunlight is its ability to stimulate the production of **vitamin D**, a hormone-like vitamin that plays an integral role in regulating metabolic processes. In this section, we will explore how sunlight enhances mitochondrial health, the relationship between vitamin D and metabolism, and safe strategies for incorporating sunlight into daily life.

How Sunlight Enhances Mitochondrial Health

Sunlight, especially **natural light in the morning**, has profound effects on our body's cellular mechanisms, particularly the mitochondria—the energy-producing powerhouses within each of our cells. Sunlight is rich in wavelengths that directly influence mitochondrial function. When sunlight enters the skin and eyes, specific wavelengths of light, particularly in the red and near-infrared spectrum, penetrate deep into the body's tissues, where they stimulate mitochondrial activity.

The process by which sunlight enhances mitochondrial function is primarily through **photobiomodulation**. Photobiomodulation occurs when the mitochondria absorb light, triggering a cascade of reactions that boost their ability to produce **adenosine triphosphate (ATP)**, the molecule responsible for energy storage and transfer in cells. ATP production is central to all cellular processes, from muscle contraction to immune function. When mitochondrial function is optimized, energy is produced more efficiently, leading to enhanced overall metabolic function. This means better endurance, faster recovery from physical activity, and a higher capacity to manage metabolic challenges, such as stress and inflammation.

Sunlight exposure also helps regulate the body's **circadian rhythm**, which influences mitochondrial health. The circadian rhythm, or our internal body clock, controls when we feel awake and when we feel tired, and it is intimately connected to how well our cells, including mitochondria, function. Early morning sunlight is particularly effective at resetting the circadian rhythm, as the blue light in the morning sky signals to the brain that it's time to wake up and start producing energy. By synchronizing your internal clock with natural light cycles, you ensure that your cells are functioning optimally throughout the day.

Exposure to natural light can also reduce **oxidative stress**, a condition caused by an imbalance between free radicals and antioxidants in the body. Excessive oxidative stress damages cells, including mitochondria, which diminishes energy production and contributes to aging and disease. Sunlight, especially red and near-infrared light, has been shown to activate certain pathways in cells that enhance their antioxidant defenses, helping the body neutralize free radicals and protect mitochondria from damage. This preservation of mitochondrial function not only improves energy production but also supports long-term metabolic health by reducing inflammation and preventing the onset of chronic conditions.

The Connection Between Vitamin D and Metabolism

One of the most well-known and vital effects of sunlight on the body is its role in stimulating the production of **vitamin D**. While it is possible to obtain vitamin D from certain foods and supplements, sunlight is the most effective natural source. When ultraviolet B (UVB) rays from the sun hit the skin, they trigger the conversion of a cholesterol derivative into vitamin D3, the active form of the vitamin. This process is crucial for many aspects of health, including bone strength, immune function, and most importantly, metabolic regulation.

Vitamin D acts more like a hormone than a traditional vitamin, and it has widespread effects on nearly every organ system in the body, particularly in maintaining **insulin sensitivity**. As we explored in Chapter 9, insulin sensitivity is critical for the regulation of blood sugar levels. When cells become resistant to insulin, it leads to impaired glucose metabolism, which can result in type 2 diabetes and other metabolic disorders. Vitamin D plays a key role in ensuring that cells remain responsive to insulin, allowing for better control of blood sugar and reducing the risk of developing insulin resistance. Studies have shown that individuals with low levels of vitamin D are at a significantly higher risk of developing type 2 diabetes, and vitamin D supplementation or adequate sun exposure can help improve glucose tolerance and metabolic efficiency.

Additionally, vitamin D is involved in the regulation of **fat metabolism**. It influences the body's ability to store and break down fat by acting on receptors in fat tissue, helping to mobilize stored fat for energy production. This not only aids in weight management but also helps maintain a balanced body composition, supporting lean muscle mass while reducing excess fat. Given the rise in obesity and related metabolic disorders, ensuring adequate vitamin D levels is a critical strategy for promoting healthy fat metabolism and preventing weight gain.

Vitamin D also plays an important role in controlling **inflammation**. Chronic inflammation is a key driver of metabolic dysfunction, contributing to conditions such as obesity, cardiovascular disease, and insulin resistance. Vitamin D helps modulate the immune system, reducing the release of pro-inflammatory cytokines while promoting anti-inflammatory pathways. This anti-inflammatory effect is particularly beneficial for metabolic health, as it helps to protect against the inflammation-driven damage to cells, including those in the liver, muscle, and adipose tissue.

The benefits of vitamin D are far-reaching, impacting everything from immune system regulation to muscle health, but its most profound effects are on metabolic processes. Ensuring sufficient vitamin D levels through regular sun exposure is not just about avoiding deficiency; it's about optimizing metabolic function and preventing the onset of serious health conditions.

Safe Ways to Maximize Sunlight Exposure

While sunlight is essential for health, it is also important to approach sun exposure safely to avoid the harmful effects of excessive ultraviolet (UV) radiation, which can lead to skin damage and increase the risk of skin cancer. The key is to strike a balance between getting enough sunlight to reap its metabolic benefits while minimizing the risks of overexposure.

For most people, **early morning or late afternoon sunlight** is the best time to be outdoors, as UV radiation is less intense during these hours. In these timeframes, you can still benefit from sunlight's positive effects on mitochondrial health and vitamin D production without the heightened risk of skin damage. Spending 15 to 30 minutes outdoors during these periods, with some skin exposed to direct sunlight, is usually sufficient to maintain adequate vitamin D levels. The exact amount of time needed can vary depending on your skin tone, location, and the time of year, but even short bursts of regular sunlight can make a significant difference.

Exposure to different parts of the body is another effective strategy. Larger areas of skin, such as the arms, legs, or back, have more surface area for absorbing UVB rays, so exposing these areas to the sun for short periods can increase vitamin D synthesis without overexposing more sensitive areas, such as the face. On days when you can't spend much time outdoors, taking a short walk in direct sunlight—especially without sunscreen or excessive clothing—can still provide enough exposure to keep your vitamin D levels in a healthy range.

For those living in regions with limited sunlight, especially during the winter months, **light therapy** or **UVB lamps** can be useful alternatives to natural sunlight. These devices mimic the beneficial effects of natural sunlight and can help maintain adequate vitamin D levels during periods of low sun exposure. However, it's essential to use these tools according to guidelines to avoid overexposure, and regular testing of vitamin D levels can help ensure that supplementation or artificial light therapy is appropriate for your needs.

Finally, it's important to stay mindful of sun exposure during peak hours (typically between 10 a.m. and 4 p.m.), when UV radiation is strongest. If you're spending extended time outdoors during these hours, wearing protective clothing, seeking shade, and using sunscreen on sensitive areas like the face and neck can help protect against the harmful effects of too much sun while still allowing you to enjoy its metabolic benefits.

7.5 Reducing EMF Exposure for Better Health

In today's world, we are constantly surrounded by technology, from smartphones and Wi-Fi routers to smart home devices and countless other forms of wireless communication. While these advancements have brought many conveniences, they also expose us to **electromagnetic fields (EMFs)**—invisible areas of energy emitted by electrical devices. As research on the effects of EMFs grows, concerns about how these fields may influence human health, particularly metabolic and cellular functions, are becoming more prevalent. Understanding the potential risks of EMF exposure and taking steps to reduce it can be a proactive way to support long-term metabolic health.

Understanding Electromagnetic Frequencies (EMFs)

EMFs are a form of non-ionizing radiation, meaning that they do not have enough energy to remove tightly bound electrons from atoms or molecules and cause ionization.

Unlike ionizing radiation, such as X-rays and gamma rays, which are known to cause direct DNA damage and increase cancer risk, non-ionizing EMFs are generally considered less harmful. However, this does not mean they are entirely without impact.

There are two main types of EMFs: **low-frequency** EMFs, such as those emitted by power lines and household electrical appliances, and **radiofrequency (RF) radiation**, which comes from wireless devices like cell phones, Wi-Fi networks, and Bluetooth devices. The concern is that, although these are low-energy waves, prolonged or excessive exposure to EMFs may have subtle, long-term effects on the body, particularly on cellular and metabolic functions.

One of the main ways in which EMFs may influence health is through their interaction with cells, specifically the **mitochondria**. As we've explored in previous chapters, mitochondria are responsible for producing energy in the form of adenosine triphosphate (ATP). Some studies suggest that EMF exposure can cause oxidative stress in cells, leading to mitochondrial dysfunction. When the mitochondria are not operating optimally, the body's energy production declines, which can affect everything from physical endurance to metabolic regulation. This has led researchers to investigate a potential link between chronic EMF exposure and metabolic disorders, including obesity, insulin resistance, and even diabetes.

In addition to the effects on mitochondria, EMF exposure may also interfere with the body's natural **electrical signals**. Our cells communicate and regulate various processes through low-frequency electrical signals, particularly in the brain and nervous system. Prolonged exposure to external electromagnetic fields could disrupt these signals, leading to imbalances in the autonomic nervous system, which controls vital functions such as digestion, heart rate, and blood sugar regulation. As we've seen in Chapter 9, maintaining hormonal and nervous system balance is essential for metabolic health, and disturbances in these systems can lead to serious metabolic consequences over time.

Although the research on EMFs is still evolving, there is enough evidence to suggest that taking measures to minimize unnecessary exposure, especially during sensitive times like sleep, could help reduce the potential risks to cellular and metabolic health.

How EMFs Disrupt Sleep and Metabolic Function

One of the most significant ways in which EMF exposure can impact health is through its effects on **sleep quality**. Sleep, as we discussed in Chapter 3, is crucial for maintaining metabolic function, and disruptions to sleep can have cascading effects on metabolism, hormone regulation, and overall health. Studies have shown that nighttime EMF exposure can interfere with the production of **melatonin**, the hormone responsible for regulating the sleep-wake cycle. Melatonin is produced by the pineal gland in response to darkness, helping the body prepare for sleep. However, exposure to EMFs—particularly RF radiation from smartphones, tablets, and Wi-Fi networks—can inhibit melatonin production, making it harder to fall asleep and stay asleep.

Reduced melatonin levels not only impair sleep but also increase oxidative stress and inflammation. Melatonin is a powerful antioxidant, and its protective effects extend beyond sleep regulation to include defending the body against cellular damage. By reducing melatonin production, EMF exposure may contribute to increased oxidative stress, which, as we've seen in previous chapters, is a major driver of metabolic dysfunction and chronic disease. Chronic oxidative stress can impair mitochondrial function, reduce energy production, and lead to insulin resistance, further complicating metabolic health.

Additionally, the blue light emitted by screens on smartphones, computers, and other devices can exacerbate these issues. Blue light has been shown to suppress melatonin even more effectively than other wavelengths of light, contributing to sleep disturbances and metabolic dysregulation. Many people are exposed to blue light and EMFs late into the evening, just when the body should be winding down and preparing for rest. This can create a cycle of poor sleep, increased stress, and disrupted metabolic function, all of which contribute to long-term health issues like weight gain, insulin resistance, and increased risk of cardiovascular disease.

Practical Steps to Minimize EMF Exposure

Given the ubiquity of EMFs in modern life, completely eliminating exposure is nearly impossible, but there are practical steps you can take to reduce your EMF burden, particularly in ways that support sleep and metabolic health.

First, consider **creating an EMF-free environment in your bedroom**. Since sleep is the time when the body undergoes repair and regeneration, reducing EMF exposure during the night can help improve sleep quality and support metabolic function. Start by removing any electronic devices, such as smartphones, tablets, and Wi-Fi routers, from the bedroom. Many people use their phones as alarms, but opting for a simple, battery-operated alarm clock can help reduce EMF exposure while still allowing you to wake up on time. If it's not possible to remove certain devices, consider turning them off or putting them in **airplane mode** to limit their EMF emissions during the night.

Reducing screen time before bed is another effective way to minimize EMF exposure and its impact on sleep. As we discussed earlier, blue light from screens can suppress melatonin production, so it's essential to limit screen use at least one hour before bedtime. Using **blue light filters** or **blue light blocking glasses** can help mitigate some of these effects if avoiding screens entirely is not feasible, but turning off devices altogether is the most effective strategy.

Another important consideration is the **placement of Wi-Fi routers** and other wireless devices in the home. Wi-Fi routers emit continuous RF radiation, which can contribute to EMF exposure throughout the day. Placing the router in a central location away from bedrooms and living areas can reduce your proximity to EMFs. Additionally, many routers have a function that allows them to be turned off at night, significantly reducing exposure while you sleep.

For those concerned about the cumulative effects of EMF exposure, **hardwiring devices** like computers and televisions with Ethernet cables instead of using wireless connections can further limit exposure. While this may seem inconvenient in a world that thrives on wireless connectivity, it can significantly reduce the EMF load in your environment, particularly for individuals who are sensitive to EMFs.

Finally, consider **grounding techniques** or **earthing**, which involve connecting with the Earth's natural electric charge by walking barefoot on grass, sand, or soil. Some proponents of grounding suggest that it helps to neutralize the positive charge that builds up in the body from exposure to EMFs. While more research is needed in this area, grounding is a simple, natural practice that may help balance the body's electrical system and promote overall well-being.

Practical Steps for a Balanced Approach to Technology

While reducing exposure to EMFs is important, it's equally essential to approach the subject with a balanced mindset. Technology plays an undeniable role in modern life, and for many people, it offers significant benefits, from connectivity to productivity. The goal should not be to create fear around EMFs but rather to use technology in a way that supports health while minimizing potential risks.

One of the simplest ways to do this is to **practice digital mindfulness**—being aware of how often you're using technology and taking regular breaks to disconnect. Spending time outdoors, engaging in physical activity, and prioritizing face-to-face interactions can help balance the time spent in front of screens and reduce overall EMF exposure. By consciously limiting the amount of time spent in high-EMF environments, you can protect your health while still enjoying the conveniences that modern technology offers.

EMF exposure is a growing concern in the digital age, and while the research is still emerging, it's clear that taking steps to reduce unnecessary exposure can benefit both metabolic and overall health. By creating a low-EMF environment during sleep, reducing screen time before bed, and being mindful of how you use technology, you can minimize the potential risks associated with EMF exposure and support better energy production, improved sleep, and long-term metabolic resilience.

Chapter 8: Mental Health and Metabolic Wellness

The connection between mental health and metabolic wellness is a critical aspect of overall well-being that is often overlooked. Stress, anxiety, and emotional imbalances can have profound effects on the body's metabolism, leading to disruptions in energy regulation, insulin sensitivity, and hormonal balance. Conversely, poor metabolic health can contribute to mood disorders and cognitive decline, creating a cycle that is difficult to break.

Mental well-being and metabolic function are intricately linked through processes such as the regulation of cortisol, the body's primary stress hormone, and the gut-brain axis, which influences both mood and metabolism. Emerging research highlights the role of stress management, mindfulness, and emotional balance in supporting metabolic health and reducing the risk of chronic diseases.

In this chapter, we will explore how mental health conditions such as chronic stress, anxiety, and depression affect metabolic processes, and vice versa. We'll also discuss strategies to manage mental and emotional stress, improve mental clarity, and enhance metabolic resilience through practices like mindfulness, gut health optimization, and stress-reduction techniques.

8.1 How Stress Impacts Metabolic Health

Stress has become a ubiquitous part of modern life, and while our bodies are equipped to handle occasional bouts of stress, chronic stress presents a far more serious challenge. The physiological response to stress is designed to be short-term, helping the body to react to immediate threats, but in today's world, many people experience prolonged periods of stress, which can wreak havoc on their metabolic health. The body's ability to regulate blood sugar, process energy efficiently, and maintain a balanced hormonal state becomes compromised when stress becomes a constant companion. In this section, we will explore the link between chronic stress and insulin resistance, how stress contributes to metabolic dysfunction, and the mind-body practices that can help manage stress to protect metabolic health.

The Link Between Chronic Stress and Insulin Resistance

When the body experiences stress, whether it's emotional, physical, or psychological, it initiates the **fight-or-flight response**, a survival mechanism that releases stress hormones such as cortisol and adrenaline. These hormones are designed to prepare the body for action, providing a quick burst of energy by mobilizing glucose (sugar) from storage to the bloodstream. This increase in blood sugar ensures that muscles have the energy they need to respond to danger. Under normal circumstances, once the stressor is gone, cortisol levels drop, and blood sugar levels return to baseline.

However, in the case of chronic stress—whether it's due to work pressure, financial concerns, relationship issues, or other long-term stressors—cortisol levels remain elevated over extended periods. This **persistent elevation of cortisol** leads to higher-than-normal blood sugar levels, which forces the pancreas to produce more insulin to help shuttle that excess sugar into cells. Over time, cells begin to become less responsive to insulin, a condition known as **insulin resistance**. As insulin resistance develops, blood sugar levels remain elevated, and the body must produce even more insulin to try to maintain normal glucose levels.

Insulin resistance is a precursor to several serious metabolic conditions, including **type 2 diabetes**, obesity, and cardiovascular disease. As we explored in Chapter 9, insulin is the key hormone responsible for regulating blood sugar, and when cells become resistant to it, the entire metabolic system suffers. Chronic stress exacerbates this condition by continuously elevating cortisol and other stress hormones, leading to prolonged periods of high blood sugar and insulin demand. Additionally, stress-induced insulin resistance can make it more difficult for individuals to lose weight, as insulin is also involved in fat storage. The more insulin present in the bloodstream, the more the body tends to store fat, particularly around the abdomen, a hallmark of **metabolic syndrome**.

Furthermore, chronic stress contributes to **dysregulation of appetite**, leading to cravings for high-calorie, carbohydrate-rich foods. This is largely driven by cortisol's influence on the body's energy regulation. When under stress, the brain seeks out fast, easily accessible sources of energy—often in the form of sugary, processed foods. These cravings are not only a response to the need for quick energy but are also part of a reward-seeking behavior initiated by stress, making it difficult to maintain a balanced, healthy diet. As we discussed in Chapter 2, nutrition plays a critical role in supporting metabolic health, and stress-induced eating patterns often lead to poor dietary choices, further compounding the effects of insulin resistance and metabolic dysfunction.

How Stress Leads to Metabolic Dysfunction

Stress is not just about its immediate effects on insulin and blood sugar; its impact on the **autonomic nervous system (ANS)** also plays a major role in long-term metabolic dysfunction. The autonomic nervous system is responsible for regulating involuntary physiological processes, including heart rate, digestion, and respiration. It is divided into two branches: the **sympathetic nervous system (SNS)**, which controls the fight-or-flight response, and the **parasympathetic nervous system (PNS)**, which governs rest and digestion.

Under chronic stress, the sympathetic nervous system is constantly activated, leading to what is commonly known as **sympathetic dominance**. In this state, the body is perpetually in a heightened state of alert, and functions that are not immediately necessary for survival, such as digestion, hormone production, and cellular repair, are downregulated. This chronic activation of the sympathetic nervous system leads to a host of metabolic problems.

When the body is in sympathetic overdrive, **digestive function is impaired**. Stress diverts blood flow away from the digestive organs to the muscles, heart, and lungs in preparation for action. Over time, this can lead to reduced nutrient absorption, slowed metabolism, and gastrointestinal issues such as irritable bowel syndrome (IBS) or leaky gut, conditions that are often linked to metabolic imbalances. Poor digestion further exacerbates metabolic dysfunction by depriving the body of the essential nutrients it needs to support energy production, repair tissues, and regulate blood sugar levels.

Cortisol directly impacts the storage of fat, particularly visceral fat—the type of fat that surrounds the organs and is associated with an increased risk of heart disease, stroke, and type 2 diabetes. Cortisol encourages the storage of excess fat in the abdominal area, contributing to the development of a "stress belly," a visible manifestation of chronic stress. This accumulation of visceral fat not only increases the risk of metabolic diseases but also produces its own inflammatory markers, perpetuating a vicious cycle of inflammation and metabolic dysfunction. Chronic inflammation, as discussed in earlier chapters, plays a central role in the development of insulin resistance, heart disease, and other metabolic conditions.

Stress disrupts the **sleep cycle**, which is critical for maintaining metabolic health. Elevated cortisol levels at night can interfere with melatonin production, leading to difficulties falling asleep or staying asleep. As we explored in Chapter 3, sleep is essential for regulating hormones, including insulin, ghrelin, and leptin, which control appetite, metabolism, and energy expenditure. A lack of restorative sleep leads to increased hunger, cravings, and further disruptions in metabolic balance.

Chronic stress also affects the **hypothalamic-pituitary-adrenal (HPA) axis**, the system responsible for controlling stress responses. Prolonged activation of the HPA axis can lead to adrenal fatigue, where the body's ability to produce cortisol becomes impaired. This results in feelings of constant exhaustion, low energy, and an inability to manage stress effectively, which compounds the body's metabolic dysfunction.

Mind-Body Practices to Manage Stress

Managing chronic stress is not just about reducing stressors; it's about cultivating resilience and teaching the body how to better respond to stress. **Mind-body practices** are among the most effective strategies for restoring balance to both the nervous system and metabolic health. These practices help activate the parasympathetic nervous system, which promotes relaxation, digestion, and healing—functions that are critical for metabolic recovery.

One of the most effective practices for managing stress is **mindfulness meditation**. Mindfulness encourages individuals to focus on the present moment, helping to break the cycle of anxious thoughts and overthinking that often accompany chronic stress. Studies have shown that mindfulness meditation can lower cortisol levels, reduce inflammation, and improve insulin sensitivity, all of which contribute to better metabolic health. Incorporating just 10 to 15 minutes of mindfulness meditation into your daily routine can help reset the nervous system and improve the body's ability to cope with stress.

Breathing exercises, such as diaphragmatic breathing or alternate nostril breathing, are another powerful tool for stress management. These exercises slow down the heart rate and promote deep relaxation, signaling to the body that it's safe to shift from the sympathetic state to the parasympathetic state. Over time, regular breathing exercises can improve heart rate variability (HRV), an indicator of how well the body adapts to stress. Higher HRV is associated with better metabolic function and a lower risk of metabolic disorders.

Physical activity is another effective way to manage stress and improve metabolic health. As we explored in Chapter 4, exercise helps to burn excess glucose, improve insulin sensitivity, and reduce cortisol levels. Activities like yoga and tai chi combine physical movement with mindful breathing, helping to lower stress while also enhancing metabolic function. Engaging in regular physical activity not only reduces the harmful effects of stress but also supports the body's energy production, making it easier to maintain a healthy metabolism.

Ensuring that you **get enough sleep** is crucial for managing stress and protecting metabolic health. Establishing a consistent sleep routine, practicing good sleep hygiene, and creating a calming bedtime ritual can help regulate cortisol levels and improve the quality of your rest. As we've seen throughout the book, sleep is foundational to metabolic health, and managing stress is key to achieving restful, restorative sleep.

8.2 The Gut-Brain Axis and Mental Well-Being

The connection between the gut and the brain is one of the most fascinating areas of emerging health research. Known as the **gut-brain axis**, this communication network between the gastrointestinal system and the brain plays a pivotal role in both mental and metabolic health. It's now widely recognized that the gut, often referred to as the "second brain," has a profound influence on our emotional well-being, mental clarity, and mood. This bidirectional relationship between the gut and the brain is mediated by the **vagus nerve**, the immune system, and the gut microbiome—a complex community of trillions of microorganisms that live in the digestive tract. In this section, we will explore how gut health affects mental clarity and mood, the role of probiotics in supporting mental health, and how to nourish the gut-brain connection through diet.

How Gut Health Affects Mental Clarity and Mood

The health of your gut significantly influences your brain function, emotional state, and cognitive performance. The gut-brain axis is an intricate system of communication that uses **neurotransmitters**, hormones, and immune signals to relay information between the two organs. One of the most critical pathways in this communication is the **vagus nerve**, which sends signals from the gut to the brain and vice versa. This means that the state of your gut—whether it's healthy or inflamed—can directly affect how you feel emotionally, as well as how clearly you think.

One of the key ways the gut influences the brain is through the production of **neurotransmitters**. Neurotransmitters are chemicals that transmit signals between nerve cells and are responsible for regulating mood, cognition, and stress responses. Remarkably, a significant portion of the body's serotonin—a neurotransmitter often referred to as the "feel-good" hormone—is produced in the gut. Approximately 90% of the body's serotonin is synthesized by gut cells and the microbes that reside there. Serotonin is critical for mood regulation, and imbalances in serotonin levels have been linked to conditions such as depression, anxiety, and mood disorders. This means that an unhealthy gut can lead to disruptions in serotonin production, potentially affecting emotional stability and mental clarity.

Additionally, the gut produces other important neurotransmitters, such as **gamma-aminobutyric acid (GABA)**, which helps calm the brain and reduce anxiety, and **dopamine**, which is involved in motivation and reward. When the gut microbiome is out of balance—often due to factors such as poor diet, stress, antibiotics, or environmental toxins—it can lead to decreased production of these key neurotransmitters, resulting in increased feelings of stress, anxiety, and brain fog. These imbalances can have a profound impact on mental health, making it harder to think clearly, concentrate, or remain emotionally stable.

Inflammation in the gut also plays a significant role in disrupting the gut-brain axis. When the gut becomes inflamed—due to a condition like **leaky gut syndrome**, poor diet, or chronic stress—**pro-inflammatory cytokines** are released into the bloodstream. These inflammatory molecules can cross the blood-brain barrier, leading to neuroinflammation. Chronic neuroinflammation has been linked to various mental health conditions, including depression, anxiety, and cognitive decline. In fact, there is growing evidence that inflammation in the gut can trigger depressive symptoms by interfering with neurotransmitter production and increasing oxidative stress in the brain.

Moreover, the **gut microbiome**—the diverse community of bacteria, viruses, and fungi that reside in the digestive tract—plays an essential role in maintaining the gut-brain connection. The composition and diversity of gut microbes can influence brain function, mood, and even the body's stress response. A healthy, balanced microbiome contributes to the production of anti-inflammatory compounds and neurotransmitters that support brain health, while an imbalanced microbiome, or **dysbiosis**, can promote inflammation and disrupt mental clarity.

The Role of Probiotics in Supporting Mental Health

Given the vital role that the gut plays in regulating mood and cognitive function, it's no surprise that **probiotics**—live beneficial bacteria—are gaining recognition for their potential to support mental health. Probiotics help to restore balance in the gut microbiome, which in turn promotes better communication between the gut and brain. Research has increasingly pointed to the use of **psychobiotics**, a subset of probiotics that specifically target the gut-brain axis, as an effective way to improve mood, reduce anxiety, and enhance mental clarity.

One of the primary ways probiotics benefit mental health is by promoting the production of **short-chain fatty acids (SCFAs)**, such as butyrate, acetate, and propionate. These fatty acids are produced when gut bacteria ferment fiber in the colon, and they have potent anti-inflammatory and neuroprotective effects. SCFAs help to strengthen the intestinal barrier, reducing gut permeability and preventing the release of inflammatory cytokines into the bloodstream. By lowering inflammation in the gut, probiotics can help mitigate the neuroinflammatory processes that contribute to depression, anxiety, and cognitive impairments.

Probiotics also influence the **hypothalamic-pituitary-adrenal (HPA) axis**, the body's central stress response system. Chronic stress can lead to dysregulation of the HPA axis, resulting in elevated cortisol levels and a heightened stress response. This, in turn, affects mood, anxiety levels, and mental clarity. Certain probiotic strains, such as **Lactobacillus rhamnosus** and **Bifidobacterium longum**, have been shown to lower cortisol levels and reduce anxiety in both animal and human studies. These psychobiotic strains modulate the HPA axis, helping to create a more balanced response to stress and supporting emotional well-being.

Another benefit of probiotics is their ability to increase **serotonin production**. As mentioned earlier, much of the body's serotonin is produced in the gut, and probiotics play a key role in this process. Studies have demonstrated that supplementing with specific strains of probiotics, such as **Lactobacillus helveticus** and **Bifidobacterium breve**, can enhance serotonin production, leading to improvements in mood and reductions in depressive symptoms.

Furthermore, probiotics help support mental health by **improving sleep quality**. The gut-brain axis also regulates sleep patterns, and an imbalanced microbiome can lead to disrupted sleep, which in turn affects mood and cognitive performance. Probiotics have been shown to improve the production of **melatonin**, a hormone that regulates the sleep-wake cycle. By promoting better sleep, probiotics indirectly support mental clarity, emotional regulation, and stress resilience.

Incorporating probiotics into your daily routine—whether through foods like yogurt, kefir, sauerkraut, or through high-quality probiotic supplements—can help maintain a healthy gut-brain axis, supporting both mental and metabolic health. Regular consumption of probiotics encourages a diverse and balanced microbiome, which plays a key role in maintaining emotional stability and cognitive function.

Nourishing the Gut-Brain Connection Through Diet

While probiotics can play an important role in supporting gut health, the overall **diet** remains a foundational aspect of maintaining a healthy gut-brain axis. Diet influences the composition of the gut microbiome, the integrity of the gut lining, and the body's inflammatory response, all of which affect mental well-being. A diet rich in nutrient-dense, whole foods can nourish both the gut and the brain, helping to optimize mental clarity, mood, and emotional stability.

One of the key nutrients for supporting the gut-brain axis is **fiber**, particularly **prebiotic fiber**, which acts as food for beneficial gut bacteria. Foods rich in prebiotics, such as garlic, onions, leeks, bananas, and asparagus, help stimulate the growth of healthy gut bacteria, enhancing the production of short-chain fatty acids that reduce inflammation and support neurotransmitter balance. By regularly consuming prebiotic-rich foods, you create an environment in the gut that fosters the production of serotonin, GABA, and other neurotransmitters that are critical for mental health.

In addition to fiber, **omega-3 fatty acids** play a crucial role in supporting both gut and brain health. Omega-3s, found in fatty fish like salmon, sardines, and mackerel, as well as in flaxseeds and walnuts, have anti-inflammatory properties that protect the gut lining and support brain function. Omega-3s help reduce inflammation in both the gut and the brain, promoting better mental clarity, improved mood, and a more resilient stress response. They also contribute to the integrity of the gut lining, preventing the development of leaky gut syndrome, which, as we've discussed, can trigger neuroinflammation and cognitive decline.

Polyphenols, a class of antioxidants found in foods such as berries, dark chocolate, green tea, and turmeric, also play a significant role in supporting the gut-brain axis. Polyphenols help nourish beneficial gut bacteria and reduce oxidative stress in both the gut and brain. By promoting the growth of healthy gut microbes and reducing inflammation, polyphenols help improve mental clarity and emotional resilience. Including polyphenol-rich foods in your daily diet is an effective way to support both gut health and cognitive function.

Finally, it's essential to limit foods that contribute to gut inflammation and dysbiosis, such as **processed sugars**, **refined carbohydrates**, and **industrial seed oils**. These foods promote the growth of harmful bacteria and increase the permeability of the gut lining, leading to inflammation that can disrupt the gut-brain axis. Instead, focus on whole, unprocessed foods that provide the nutrients needed to maintain a balanced gut microbiome and support mental health.

8.3 The Effects of Anxiety and Depression on Metabolism

The connection between mental health and physical health is far more profound than we once understood. Anxiety and depression, two of the most common mental health conditions worldwide, can have a significant impact on metabolic function. While these disorders primarily affect mood, thoughts, and emotions, they also trigger biological changes that directly influence metabolism, energy regulation, and overall health. In this section, we'll explore how anxiety and depression alter energy production, how these mental health conditions contribute to metabolic dysfunction, and strategies to break the cycle and restore balance.

How Mental Health Conditions Alter Energy Production

When the body experiences anxiety or depression, it isn't just the mind that's affected; the entire body is involved in the response. Both anxiety and depression initiate physiological changes that influence how the body processes and produces energy. These mental health conditions often trigger a heightened **stress response**, leading to an overproduction of **cortisol**, the body's primary stress hormone. Elevated cortisol levels can disrupt numerous metabolic processes, from insulin sensitivity to fat storage.

In the case of **anxiety**, the body is frequently in a state of heightened alert, activating the **sympathetic nervous system**—the part of the nervous system responsible for the fight-or-flight response. This constant state of readiness causes an increase in heart rate, blood pressure, and the release of glucose into the bloodstream to provide immediate energy. While this may be beneficial in the short term, chronic anxiety keeps the body in this heightened state, leading to a sustained release of glucose and insulin, which can eventually result in **insulin resistance**. Insulin resistance, as we've seen in previous chapters, can contribute to the development of metabolic conditions such as type 2 diabetes and obesity.

Depression, on the other hand, often leads to **chronic fatigue** and low energy, despite metabolic changes that might suggest otherwise. Depression can suppress physical activity and reduce motivation, which decreases energy expenditure. This sedentary behavior combined with metabolic disruptions—such as changes in appetite and sleep patterns—can lead to an imbalance between energy intake and output. Over time, this imbalance can contribute to weight gain, insulin resistance, and a host of other metabolic issues.

Additionally, depression is associated with a reduction in **mitochondrial function**, the cellular organelles responsible for producing energy. When mitochondrial function is impaired, the body's ability to produce **adenosine triphosphate (ATP)**—the energy currency of the cells—declines. This decrease in energy production can further exacerbate feelings of fatigue and lethargy commonly experienced in depression. Moreover, mitochondrial dysfunction increases oxidative stress, which damages cells and contributes to the inflammation that is often seen in both mental health disorders and metabolic diseases.

Another factor that ties mental health conditions to metabolism is **sleep disruption**. Anxiety and depression frequently lead to sleep disturbances, including insomnia or excessive sleeping. As we've discussed in Chapter 3, poor sleep can significantly disrupt metabolic function by impairing insulin sensitivity, increasing hunger hormones such as **ghrelin**, and reducing satiety hormones such as **leptin**. This hormonal imbalance promotes overeating and weight gain, further contributing to metabolic dysfunction.

The Cycle Between Poor Mental Health and Metabolic Dysfunction

The relationship between mental health and metabolism is not one-sided; just as anxiety and depression can negatively impact metabolism, metabolic dysfunction can, in turn, worsen mental health. This creates a **vicious cycle**, where each condition feeds into the other, making it more challenging to break free from the effects of both.

One of the key ways that metabolic dysfunction exacerbates mental health conditions is through **inflammation**. Chronic inflammation, which is commonly associated with metabolic disorders such as obesity and type 2 diabetes, can contribute to the development of anxiety and depression. Inflammation triggers the release of pro-inflammatory cytokines, which can cross the **blood-brain barrier** and alter brain function, contributing to mood disorders. In fact, research has shown that individuals with higher levels of inflammatory markers are more likely to experience symptoms of depression and anxiety.

Additionally, metabolic conditions such as obesity can impact **neurotransmitter function**, particularly serotonin, which plays a critical role in mood regulation. As we explored in Chapter 8.2, the gut is a major producer of serotonin, and metabolic conditions that disrupt gut health—such as insulin resistance or an unhealthy diet—can interfere with serotonin production, leading to mood imbalances.

Moreover, individuals with metabolic dysfunction often experience **poor body image** and **reduced self-esteem**, particularly when weight gain is involved. This negative self-perception can increase feelings of anxiety and depression, further perpetuating the cycle. As the mental health conditions worsen, individuals may engage in **unhealthy coping mechanisms**, such as emotional eating or avoiding physical activity, which only exacerbates metabolic dysfunction.

Another major factor in the cycle between mental health and metabolism is **stress eating**. Individuals with anxiety and depression are more likely to turn to **comfort foods**—which are typically high in sugar, unhealthy fats, and refined carbohydrates—as a way to cope with their emotional state. These foods may temporarily improve mood by increasing dopamine levels, but in the long term, they contribute to metabolic dysfunction by promoting weight gain, insulin resistance, and inflammation.

This cycle between poor mental health and metabolic dysfunction highlights the importance of addressing both aspects simultaneously in order to achieve lasting improvement in overall well-being. By breaking the cycle and treating the root causes of both mental and metabolic health issues, individuals can restore balance and improve their quality of life.

Strategies to Break the Cycle and Restore Balance

Breaking the cycle between anxiety, depression, and metabolic dysfunction requires a **holistic approach** that addresses both mental and physical health. While conventional treatments such as **therapy** and **medication** are effective for managing anxiety and depression, incorporating lifestyle changes that support metabolic health can significantly enhance treatment outcomes.

One of the most effective strategies for improving both mental and metabolic health is **physical activity**. Regular exercise has been shown to reduce symptoms of anxiety and depression by increasing the production of endorphins and serotonin, which improve mood and reduce stress. Exercise also improves insulin sensitivity, enhances mitochondrial function, and reduces inflammation, all of which contribute to better metabolic health. Engaging in physical activity—even light activities like walking or yoga—can have profound benefits for both mental well-being and metabolism.

Nutrition also plays a crucial role in breaking the cycle of mental and metabolic dysfunction. As we've discussed in previous chapters, a diet rich in whole, nutrient-dense foods such as vegetables, fruits, lean proteins, and healthy fats can support both brain and body function. Incorporating foods that are high in **omega-3 fatty acids**, such as salmon, flaxseeds, and walnuts, can help reduce inflammation and improve brain function. Additionally, limiting refined carbohydrates and sugar can prevent spikes in blood sugar and insulin levels, which are linked to both metabolic dysfunction and mood disorders.

Mind-body practices, such as **meditation, deep breathing**, and **progressive muscle relaxation**, can help reduce the physiological effects of stress, lowering cortisol levels and improving both mental clarity and metabolic function. These practices promote relaxation and improve resilience to stress, helping to break the cycle of anxiety and depression that contributes to metabolic dysfunction.

Another important strategy is to ensure adequate **sleep**. Improving sleep hygiene—such as establishing a regular bedtime routine, limiting screen time before bed, and creating a dark, quiet sleep environment—can improve both mental and metabolic health. Restorative sleep helps regulate the hormones that control hunger, satiety, and stress, reducing the likelihood of stress eating and improving insulin sensitivity.

Social support is critical for breaking the cycle of anxiety, depression, and metabolic dysfunction. Individuals who have strong social connections are more likely to engage in healthy behaviors, such as regular exercise and nutritious eating, and are less likely to experience chronic stress or feelings of isolation. Cultivating relationships with supportive friends, family members, or participating in support groups can provide emotional encouragement and accountability, helping individuals stay on track with their mental and physical health goals.

8.4 The Power of Mindfulness in Improving Metabolic Health

Mindfulness has been recognized as a powerful tool for improving mental clarity, emotional regulation, and overall well-being. However, what many people may not realize is that practicing mindfulness can also have a profound impact on **metabolic health**. The mind and body are intimately connected, and the ways in which we manage stress, regulate emotions, and stay present in the moment can directly influence key metabolic processes such as **blood sugar regulation, hormone balance**, and **inflammation**. In this section, we will explore how mindfulness affects blood sugar and cortisol levels, techniques to integrate mindfulness into daily life, and the long-term benefits of mental clarity on physical health.

How Mindfulness Affects Blood Sugar and Cortisol Levels

At the core of the connection between mindfulness and metabolic health is the **stress response**. When we experience stress—whether due to external factors like work deadlines or internal stressors such as negative thought patterns—our bodies release **cortisol**, the primary stress hormone. While cortisol is essential for survival, helping the body mobilize energy and respond to threats, chronically elevated cortisol levels can lead to **metabolic dysfunction**.

Cortisol triggers the release of **glucose** (sugar) into the bloodstream to provide quick energy. This is useful in short-term situations but can become problematic when stress is prolonged or frequent. Elevated blood sugar levels increase the demand for insulin, the hormone responsible for moving glucose into cells. Over time, chronic stress can contribute to **insulin resistance**, a condition where cells become less responsive to insulin, leading to high blood sugar levels. Insulin resistance is a precursor to **type 2 diabetes**, obesity, and other metabolic disorders.

Mindfulness, through its focus on cultivating a calm and present state of mind, has been shown to lower cortisol levels and improve blood sugar regulation. **Mindfulness-based stress reduction (MBSR)** programs and similar practices have demonstrated the ability to reduce the body's stress response, leading to more balanced cortisol levels. By lowering cortisol, mindfulness helps reduce the frequency and intensity of stress-related blood sugar spikes, allowing the body to maintain **better insulin sensitivity** and prevent the onset of metabolic disorders.

Moreover, mindfulness improves the body's ability to handle fluctuations in blood sugar. Chronic stress can create a cycle where high cortisol leads to blood sugar spikes, followed by insulin surges, which then result in energy crashes and cravings for high-sugar or high-fat foods. This cycle often contributes to **emotional eating**, weight gain, and further metabolic imbalance. Practicing mindfulness helps break this cycle by teaching individuals to become more aware of their emotional states and triggers for unhealthy eating habits. By becoming more conscious of how stress influences food choices, individuals can make better dietary decisions, stabilizing blood sugar and improving overall metabolic health.

Another critical way mindfulness impacts metabolic health is through its ability to lower **inflammation**. As we've discussed in previous chapters, chronic inflammation is a major driver of metabolic dysfunction, contributing to conditions such as insulin resistance, obesity, and cardiovascular disease. Stress is a key contributor to inflammation, and cortisol plays a role in regulating the immune response. When cortisol levels remain elevated for extended periods, it can dysregulate the immune system, leading to increased production of pro-inflammatory cytokines. By reducing stress and cortisol levels, mindfulness helps to regulate inflammation, protecting the body from the harmful effects of chronic stress and promoting better metabolic function.

Techniques to Integrate Mindfulness Into Daily Life

One of the most appealing aspects of mindfulness is that it can be practiced anywhere, at any time, making it a flexible and accessible tool for improving both mental and metabolic health. For individuals new to mindfulness, the idea of sitting in meditation for long periods can seem daunting. However, mindfulness is not limited to traditional meditation; it can be integrated into daily life through simple, intentional practices.

Mindful breathing is one of the easiest ways to begin incorporating mindfulness into your routine. It involves focusing on the breath as it moves in and out of the body, anchoring the mind in the present moment. By paying attention to the natural rhythm of your breath, you can reduce anxiety and stress, which in turn helps regulate cortisol levels. A simple technique is **diaphragmatic breathing**—breathing deeply into the belly rather than the chest—which helps activate the parasympathetic nervous system and promotes relaxation. Practicing mindful breathing for just a few minutes a day can have a calming effect on the mind and body, supporting more balanced metabolic function.

Another effective technique is **mindful eating**. Many people eat quickly or mindlessly, often distracted by work, television, or other activities. This can lead to overeating, poor digestion, and metabolic strain. Mindful eating encourages you to slow down, savor each bite, and pay attention to the sensations of hunger and fullness. By being fully present during meals, you become more attuned to your body's signals, making it easier to stop eating when you are satisfied rather than when you are overly full. This practice not only helps regulate blood sugar levels by preventing overeating but also improves digestion and nutrient absorption, key components of metabolic health.

Body scanning is another form of mindfulness that can help improve both mental and physical well-being. This practice involves mentally scanning each part of the body, starting from the feet and moving upward, paying attention to areas of tension or discomfort. The goal is to become more aware of how stress affects the body and to release any tension you may be holding. Body scanning can be particularly effective for managing chronic stress, as it encourages a deeper connection between the mind and body, helping to alleviate physical symptoms of stress, such as muscle tension, headaches, or digestive issues.

For those who prefer more active forms of mindfulness, practices such as **yoga** or **tai chi** are excellent ways to integrate mindfulness with movement. These activities focus on synchronizing breath with movement, cultivating awareness of the body's sensations and the mind's reactions. By practicing mindful movement, you can lower stress, improve flexibility and balance, and enhance metabolic health by promoting better circulation and energy regulation.

To incorporate mindfulness into your day, it's helpful to start small. For example, you could begin with five minutes of mindful breathing in the morning or a short body scan before bed. Over time, as you become more comfortable with the practice, you can gradually increase the duration of your mindfulness sessions or add new techniques. The key is consistency—regular mindfulness practice is what leads to long-term benefits.

Long-Term Benefits of Mental Clarity on Physical Health

The long-term benefits of mindfulness extend well beyond reducing stress and improving blood sugar regulation. By cultivating mental clarity and emotional balance, mindfulness sets the foundation for sustained physical health and well-being. One of the most significant long-term benefits is the promotion of **hormonal balance**. As we explored in Chapter 9, hormones play a critical role in regulating metabolism, appetite, and energy production. By managing stress and reducing cortisol levels through mindfulness, you help prevent hormonal imbalances that can lead to weight gain, insulin resistance, and other metabolic disorders.

Mindfulness also supports **better sleep**, which is essential for maintaining metabolic health. Poor sleep is often linked to elevated cortisol levels, insulin resistance, and increased appetite, particularly for sugary or high-calorie foods. Practicing mindfulness before bed—such as through mindful breathing or a body scan—can help quiet the mind, promote relaxation, and improve sleep quality. Over time, improved sleep leads to more balanced metabolic function, better energy levels, and enhanced overall well-being.

Another long-term benefit of mindfulness is its ability to reduce **emotional eating**. Emotional eating is a common response to stress, anxiety, or boredom, and it often involves consuming high-calorie, low-nutrient foods that contribute to weight gain and metabolic dysfunction. By practicing mindfulness, individuals can become more aware of their emotional triggers and learn to respond to them in healthier ways. Instead of reaching for food as a coping mechanism, mindfulness teaches you to observe your emotions without judgment, making it easier to choose more nourishing and balanced responses to stress.

Moreover, mindfulness improves **focus and decision-making**, which are critical for making healthier lifestyle choices. When the mind is clear and calm, it becomes easier to prioritize self-care activities such as exercise, balanced eating, and stress management. Over time, these positive habits lead to better metabolic health, improved weight management, and a reduced risk of developing chronic diseases.

Finally, mindfulness promotes a sense of **resilience** and **emotional regulation**, helping individuals navigate life's challenges without becoming overwhelmed by stress. This emotional resilience not only protects mental health but also supports the body's ability to adapt to metabolic stressors. Whether it's dealing with the demands of work, managing family responsibilities, or coping with health challenges, mindfulness equips individuals with the tools they need to maintain balance and well-being, both mentally and physically.

8.5 Managing Burnout: Reversing the Effects on Metabolic Health

Burnout has become a widespread issue, affecting not only mental health but also physical well-being. It doesn't just exhaust our emotional reserves—it takes a serious toll on our metabolic system, too. The feeling of constant fatigue, coupled with the physical effects of prolonged stress, can disrupt the body's ability to regulate energy and manage stress. This leads to a cascade of health issues, from insulin resistance to weight gain and inflammation. To truly understand how burnout affects our metabolism and to explore how we can restore balance, it's important to address both the mental and physical aspects.

The Metabolic Toll of Chronic Fatigue and Burnout

When we think of burnout, we typically associate it with mental exhaustion. However, the physical effects of burnout are just as significant, if not more so. Prolonged stress overactivates the **hypothalamic-pituitary-adrenal (HPA) axis**, flooding the body with cortisol. Initially, this stress hormone helps the body cope with demands by releasing glucose into the bloodstream, providing a quick source of energy. However, this short-term survival mechanism backfires when stress becomes chronic. Constantly elevated cortisol levels lead to **insulin resistance**, a condition where the body's cells stop responding efficiently to insulin, resulting in persistently high blood sugar levels.

Over time, insulin resistance can develop into more serious metabolic conditions, such as **type 2 diabetes** and **metabolic syndrome**. As we discussed earlier in Chapter 9, the body's ability to regulate blood sugar is crucial for maintaining overall health. Yet burnout impairs this regulatory system, pushing the body toward metabolic dysfunction. Moreover, chronic stress doesn't just impact insulin sensitivity—it also leads to **visceral fat accumulation**, particularly in the abdominal area, further increasing the risk of cardiovascular diseases.

But the story doesn't end there. Burnout also wreaks havoc on **mitochondrial function**—the powerhouses of our cells. These tiny organelles are responsible for producing the energy needed for every cellular process. In individuals experiencing chronic fatigue, mitochondrial function declines, resulting in lower energy production. This lack of energy manifests not only as mental fatigue but also as physical exhaustion, making it difficult for the body to repair and rejuvenate.

Imagine a car running on empty—constantly demanding energy from a drained system leaves you vulnerable to illness, weight gain, and even cognitive decline. And with **chronic inflammation** on the rise, driven by persistent stress and poor metabolic health, the body faces a constant internal battle that further weakens its defenses.

Rebuilding Resilience and Energy After Burnout

So how do we reverse these effects? Healing from burnout requires a thoughtful and holistic approach—one that considers both the mind and body. It starts with acknowledging the imbalance and making gradual changes to restore energy and metabolic function.

Rest is a critical piece of the puzzle. It might seem obvious, but it's often the most overlooked part of recovery. True rest isn't just about sleep (though that's essential); it's about creating space in your life to recharge mentally and physically. **Sleep hygiene** is the first step. Regular sleep patterns help reset the body's natural circadian rhythm, a key regulator of both cortisol and insulin levels. A consistent bedtime, free of screens and distractions, can work wonders in supporting hormonal balance. Restful sleep allows the adrenal glands, which have been overworked by stress, to recover.

Nutrition also plays a pivotal role in restoring energy levels. A diet rich in **whole foods**, particularly those high in antioxidants and healthy fats, helps to reduce inflammation and support mitochondrial repair. Foods like leafy greens, fatty fish, nuts, and seeds provide the nutrients necessary to restore cellular function. In addition to dietary changes, certain **adaptogenic herbs**, such as ashwagandha and rhodiola, can support the body's stress response by balancing cortisol levels. These herbs have been used for centuries to help the body adapt to stress, making them valuable allies in the fight against burnout.

Physical activity, while important, should be approached carefully during recovery. Intense exercise can further tax an already overworked system. Instead, focus on **gentle, restorative movements** such as yoga, tai chi, or walking. These activities not only help rebuild physical strength but also encourage relaxation and mindfulness. Reconnecting with the body in this way helps restore the parasympathetic nervous system, which is responsible for calming the body after stress.

And let's not forget the **power of mindfulness**. As we discussed in Chapter 8.4, mindfulness practices can dramatically reduce cortisol levels and improve emotional regulation. Techniques like meditation, mindful breathing, and even journaling can help bring awareness to the stressors in your life and create space to manage them more effectively. Mindfulness allows you to stay grounded in the present, reducing the tendency to spiral into stress-induced overdrive. This calm state helps the body regulate itself, improving both mental clarity and metabolic health.

Preventing Burnout in the Future

After experiencing burnout, it's crucial to be mindful of how to keep it from returning. Catching early warning signs—whether it's feeling chronically fatigued, struggling to focus, or noticing physical discomfort like headaches or stomach issues—can help you take action before stress spirals out of control. The small adjustments you make today could be what saves you from burnout later on.

One of the most effective ways to stay resilient is to build intentional **self-care** practices into your daily routine. Self-care doesn't have to be elaborate; even a few moments of quiet reflection, a short walk outside, or simply pausing to breathe deeply can make a meaningful difference. These moments act as buffers, helping your body and mind stay in sync rather than letting stress accumulate.

Equally important is learning how to **set boundaries**. Many people find themselves burnt out because they've said "yes" to too many obligations. It's often difficult to decline requests at work or in personal relationships, but doing so is essential for protecting your energy. By managing your commitments wisely, you give yourself the space to recharge. The ability to say "no" when needed isn't just about prioritizing tasks—it's about valuing your well-being.

Along with managing external demands, keeping a routine that includes regular **physical movement** is key. It doesn't have to be strenuous exercise—just consistent activity that keeps your body engaged. Moving throughout the day helps maintain a stable metabolism and keeps energy levels up. Paired with a **nutritious diet**, which provides the fuel your body needs to handle stress efficiently, these habits form the backbone of a healthy, sustainable lifestyle.

Creating opportunities for **mental and emotional rest** is just as important. Whether through mindfulness, creative expression, or engaging in hobbies you love, finding ways to nurture your mind ensures you can better navigate the stresses that come your way. The more proactive you are in supporting both your mental and physical health, the less likely you are to fall into the cycle of burnout again.

Taking control of stress and fatigue doesn't just get you back on track—it builds a stronger foundation for lasting well-being.

Chapter 9: Hormonal Balance and Metabolic Health

Hormones are the body's messengers, playing a pivotal role in regulating metabolism, energy levels, and overall health. When hormone levels become imbalanced, it can lead to significant metabolic dysfunctions, including weight gain, insulin resistance, fatigue, and other chronic conditions. Hormonal imbalances are often the result of stress, poor nutrition, environmental toxins, and age-related changes.

Key hormones such as insulin, cortisol, thyroid hormones, and sex hormones (estrogen and testosterone) have a profound impact on how the body processes energy, burns fat, and regulates blood sugar. When these hormones are not in harmony, metabolic processes can become inefficient, leading to a range of health issues.

In this chapter, we will examine how hormonal balance affects metabolic health, focusing on common issues like insulin resistance, thyroid dysfunction, and hormonal imbalances related to stress and aging. We will explore natural approaches to rebalance hormones through lifestyle interventions, diet, and stress management to restore metabolic health and well-being.

9.1 The Role of Insulin and Blood Sugar Regulation

Insulin plays a central role in how the body processes and uses energy. It's one of the most important hormones regulating metabolism, yet imbalances in insulin function are at the core of many chronic diseases. Understanding how **insulin resistance** develops and why it's so harmful to metabolic health is critical for anyone looking to optimize their overall well-being. Insulin's primary function is to help cells absorb glucose from the bloodstream, but when the body becomes resistant to insulin's effects, a cascade of metabolic issues ensue.

How Insulin Resistance Affects Overall Health

Insulin resistance occurs when the body's cells no longer respond properly to insulin, requiring the pancreas to produce more and more of the hormone to manage blood sugar levels. Initially, the pancreas compensates by overproducing insulin, but over time, this leads to **beta-cell dysfunction**—the pancreatic cells that produce insulin become exhausted and unable to keep up with demand. This ultimately results in elevated blood sugar levels, a condition known as **hyperglycemia**.

This persistent elevation in blood glucose has far-reaching consequences on the body. **Type 2 diabetes** is one of the most well-known outcomes of insulin resistance, but the impact extends beyond that. Chronically high blood sugar and insulin levels promote **inflammation** throughout the body, leading to damage in tissues and organs. This inflammation can accelerate the development of cardiovascular disease, impair kidney function, and damage nerve cells, increasing the risk of complications like neuropathy and impaired vision.

Another key effect of insulin resistance is its role in promoting **fat storage**, particularly in the abdominal area. As the body becomes resistant to insulin, it shifts from burning fat for fuel to storing it, especially around the visceral organs. This type of fat, called **visceral fat**, is particularly dangerous because it contributes to further metabolic dysregulation and inflammation, creating a vicious cycle. As visceral fat increases, it releases **pro-inflammatory cytokines** that worsen insulin resistance, leading to a greater risk of developing metabolic syndrome and other chronic conditions such as heart disease and stroke.

The connection between **insulin resistance and cognitive decline** is also becoming more evident. The brain requires a steady supply of glucose to function optimally, and when insulin resistance develops, the brain's ability to use glucose efficiently diminishes. This has been linked to an increased risk of **Alzheimer's disease** and other forms of dementia. Some researchers even refer to Alzheimer's as "type 3 diabetes" because of the role that insulin resistance and poor glucose metabolism play in its development.

The Connection Between Blood Sugar Spikes and Chronic Diseases

Frequent blood sugar spikes—caused by consuming high amounts of refined carbohydrates, sugary snacks, or large meals—are a precursor to insulin resistance. When blood sugar rises sharply, the pancreas responds by releasing a large amount of insulin to bring glucose levels back down. Over time, this repeated surge in insulin production wears down the body's ability to maintain normal blood sugar levels, contributing to **insulin resistance** and other metabolic issues.

Each time blood sugar spikes, it triggers a cascade of harmful effects in the body. **Oxidative stress**, for example, occurs when there is an imbalance between free radicals (molecules that can damage cells) and antioxidants. Blood sugar spikes lead to the production of more free radicals, damaging blood vessels, tissues, and organs. This oxidative damage accelerates the aging process and increases the risk of chronic conditions such as cardiovascular disease, kidney damage, and neuropathy.

The process of **glycation**—where excess glucose molecules bind to proteins in the body, forming **advanced glycation end-products (AGEs)**—also contributes to disease progression. AGEs cause stiffening and thickening of tissues, which can impair the function of blood vessels and organs. High levels of AGEs are associated with the complications of diabetes, such as kidney disease, retinal damage, and reduced elasticity in blood vessels, all of which can lead to serious health problems over time.

In addition to these effects, frequent blood sugar spikes are closely linked to **inflammation**. Inflammatory responses triggered by high blood sugar contribute to the development of **atherosclerosis**—the hardening of the arteries—which is a major risk factor for heart attacks and strokes. This is why individuals with diabetes or prediabetes are at significantly higher risk for cardiovascular events.

One of the more subtle but important impacts of blood sugar spikes is how they affect **mood and cognitive function**. After a sharp rise in blood sugar, there is often a subsequent crash, where blood sugar levels drop rapidly, leading to feelings of fatigue, irritability, and difficulty concentrating. Over time, these fluctuations can impair mental clarity and contribute to mood disorders such as anxiety and depression.

Simple Strategies to Stabilize Blood Sugar Levels

Fortunately, stabilizing blood sugar levels is achievable through relatively simple, sustainable lifestyle adjustments. The key is focusing on **steady energy** rather than dramatic fluctuations in glucose and insulin. This can be accomplished by making strategic changes in diet, exercise, and daily habits.

Balancing macronutrients at each meal is one of the most effective ways to avoid blood sugar spikes. Including protein, healthy fats, and fiber alongside carbohydrates helps slow down the absorption of glucose, leading to a more gradual rise in blood sugar. For example, pairing a serving of whole grains with lean protein (such as chicken or fish) and healthy fats (like avocado or olive oil) results in a slower, more controlled release of glucose into the bloodstream, preventing the sharp spikes that contribute to insulin resistance.

Another simple but powerful tool for stabilizing blood sugar is practicing **portion control**. Large meals place a heavier demand on insulin production, increasing the risk of blood sugar spikes. By eating smaller, more frequent meals, you can better manage your blood sugar throughout the day. **Intermittent fasting**, as discussed in Chapter 2.4, is another effective approach to help regulate blood sugar levels by giving the body extended periods without glucose intake, allowing insulin levels to remain stable.

Exercise plays a crucial role in improving insulin sensitivity. Even moderate physical activity, such as walking or light resistance training, helps muscles use glucose more efficiently. After a meal, taking a brief walk can help lower blood sugar levels by enhancing glucose uptake in muscle cells. Over time, regular exercise can significantly improve the body's response to insulin, reducing the risk of developing insulin resistance.

Incorporating foods with a **low glycemic index (GI)** can also prevent blood sugar spikes. Low-GI foods are digested and absorbed more slowly, leading to a gradual increase in blood sugar. Foods like legumes, whole grains, non-starchy vegetables, and most fruits are good choices for maintaining stable glucose levels. On the other hand, avoiding refined sugars and highly processed foods is critical for blood sugar control. These foods are absorbed quickly and cause sharp spikes in blood glucose.

Hydration also plays an important role. Drinking enough water helps the kidneys flush out excess sugar through urine, supporting more stable blood sugar levels. Even mild dehydration can raise blood sugar levels, so maintaining proper hydration throughout the day is essential.

Lastly, managing **stress** is a crucial, often overlooked factor in blood sugar regulation. As we explored in earlier chapters, stress triggers the release of cortisol, which increases blood sugar levels as part of the body's fight-or-flight response. Incorporating stress-reduction techniques such as mindfulness, yoga, or deep breathing can help mitigate cortisol's impact on glucose levels, keeping blood sugar more stable over time.

9.2 Thyroid Health and Metabolic Function

The thyroid gland plays a vital role in regulating metabolism, influencing how quickly or slowly the body burns calories, processes energy, and maintains overall metabolic function. This small, butterfly-shaped gland located in the neck produces hormones that are essential for numerous physiological processes, including energy production, temperature regulation, and the balance of other hormones. When the thyroid is not functioning properly, the body's metabolism can become either sluggish or overactive, leading to a range of health issues. In this section, we'll explore how thyroid function impacts metabolism, common thyroid disorders, and strategies to support thyroid health.

How the Thyroid Gland Regulates Metabolism

The primary hormones produced by the thyroid are **triiodothyronine (T3)** and **thyroxine (T4)**. These hormones control the body's **basal metabolic rate (BMR)**—the rate at which the body uses energy while at rest. Essentially, T3 and T4 determine how efficiently your body converts food into energy and how fast or slow your metabolism operates. These hormones also help regulate body temperature, heart rate, and protein synthesis, all of which are crucial for maintaining metabolic balance.

The production of thyroid hormones is regulated by the **hypothalamus** and the **pituitary gland** in the brain. When the body needs more thyroid hormones, the hypothalamus releases **thyrotropin-releasing hormone (TRH)**, which signals the pituitary gland to release **thyroid-stimulating hormone (TSH)**. TSH then prompts the thyroid to produce and release T3 and T4. This feedback loop is essential for keeping the body's metabolic processes stable.

When thyroid hormone levels are within a healthy range, the metabolism functions optimally, ensuring that the body can maintain energy balance. However, when the thyroid gland produces too much or too little of these hormones, it can lead to metabolic disorders such as **hypothyroidism** or **hyperthyroidism**.

Common Thyroid Disorders and Their Symptoms

One of the most common thyroid conditions affecting metabolism is **hypothyroidism**—a condition in which the thyroid does not produce enough T3 and T4 hormones. Hypothyroidism slows down the body's metabolic processes, leading to symptoms such as **fatigue**, **weight gain**, **cold intolerance**, **dry skin**, and **constipation**. The reduced metabolic rate means that the body burns fewer calories, making it easier to gain weight even with a normal diet. Individuals with hypothyroidism often struggle with energy levels and may feel sluggish or mentally foggy throughout the day.

Hashimoto's thyroiditis, an autoimmune disorder, is the leading cause of hypothyroidism. In Hashimoto's, the immune system mistakenly attacks the thyroid gland, causing inflammation and impairing its ability to produce thyroid hormones. This condition develops gradually, and symptoms may be mild at first, but over time, it can significantly impact metabolic health.

On the opposite end of the spectrum is **hyperthyroidism**, a condition where the thyroid produces too much T3 and T4. This condition speeds up metabolism, often leading to **unintended weight loss**, **increased appetite**, **nervousness**, **rapid heartbeat**, and **insomnia**. In hyperthyroidism, the body's processes run in overdrive, and while this might seem advantageous for weight loss, it can actually be harmful, as it places undue stress on the cardiovascular system and other organs.

One of the most common causes of hyperthyroidism is **Graves' disease**, another autoimmune disorder in which the immune system overstimulates the thyroid gland, causing it to produce excess hormones. While hyperthyroidism is less common than hypothyroidism, it can lead to serious complications, including **atrial fibrillation**, **osteoporosis**, and **thyroid storm**—a life-threatening condition characterized by extremely high thyroid hormone levels.

Both conditions can have significant impacts on **insulin sensitivity** and **fat metabolism**, further complicating an individual's ability to maintain a healthy weight and metabolic balance.

Nutritional and Lifestyle Interventions for Thyroid Health

Supporting thyroid health is crucial for maintaining overall metabolic function. Several lifestyle and dietary interventions can help optimize thyroid hormone production and protect against thyroid-related metabolic issues. While some individuals may require medication to manage thyroid conditions, there are many steps you can take to improve thyroid function naturally.

Iodine is a critical nutrient for thyroid hormone production, as T3 and T4 are made from iodine molecules. Without sufficient iodine, the thyroid cannot produce adequate hormones, leading to hypothyroidism. Iodine deficiency is relatively rare in countries where iodized salt is common, but it's important to ensure you're getting enough iodine through food sources like **seaweed, fish, dairy products**, and **iodized salt**. However, excessive iodine intake can also disrupt thyroid function, so balance is key.

Selenium is another essential mineral that plays a role in thyroid hormone metabolism. Selenium helps convert T4, the inactive form of thyroid hormone, into T3, the active form that the body uses for energy. Foods rich in selenium, such as **Brazil nuts**, **tuna, eggs**, and **sunflower seeds**, can support healthy thyroid function and reduce the risk of thyroid-related metabolic issues.

Zinc is also important for thyroid health, as it supports the production of TSH, the hormone that signals the thyroid to release T3 and T4. Zinc-rich foods like **oysters**, **pumpkin seeds**, and **beef** can enhance thyroid function and support metabolism.

In addition to focusing on specific nutrients, it's essential to maintain a **balanced diet** that includes a variety of whole foods. As we discussed in Chapter 2, a diet rich in vegetables, fruits, lean proteins, and healthy fats supports not only thyroid health but overall metabolic function. Avoiding processed foods and refined sugars, which can contribute to inflammation and disrupt hormone balance, is also critical.

Another important factor in supporting thyroid health is **stress management**. Chronic stress, as we've seen in earlier chapters, can disrupt the HPA axis and negatively affect thyroid function. High levels of cortisol, the body's primary stress hormone, interfere with the conversion of T4 to T3, leading to imbalances in thyroid hormone levels.

Incorporating stress-reduction techniques such as **meditation**, **yoga**, and **deep breathing** can help regulate cortisol levels and support healthy thyroid function.

Regular **physical activity** is also important for maintaining a healthy metabolism and supporting thyroid function. Exercise stimulates the production of thyroid hormones and improves the body's sensitivity to them. However, it's important to avoid overexertion, especially for individuals with thyroid conditions, as excessive exercise can elevate cortisol levels and further disrupt thyroid function.

Finally, **regular thyroid screenings** are essential for anyone at risk of thyroid dysfunction, especially those with a family history of thyroid disorders or autoimmune conditions. By monitoring thyroid hormone levels through blood tests, you can catch potential imbalances early and take steps to manage them before they lead to more serious metabolic issues.

9.3 Hormonal Imbalances and Weight Gain

Weight gain and difficulty managing weight are often blamed on poor diet or lack of exercise, but hormonal imbalances can also play a significant role. Hormones regulate almost every aspect of how your body processes food, stores fat, and uses energy. When these hormones are out of balance, even a healthy lifestyle may not be enough to keep weight in check. In this section, we'll explore how hormones such as **estrogen**, **testosterone**, and others influence fat distribution, how hormonal imbalances lead to metabolic dysfunction, and ways to rebalance these hormones to support healthy weight management.

The Role of Estrogen and Testosterone in Fat Distribution

Estrogen and testosterone are two of the primary hormones that regulate fat storage and muscle mass in both men and women. While they're often associated with sexual and reproductive health, these hormones also have significant effects on metabolism and body composition.

Estrogen, the primary female sex hormone, is responsible for regulating fat distribution, particularly around the hips and thighs in women. This fat storage pattern, known as **gynoid fat distribution**, is considered less harmful than the visceral fat that accumulates around the abdomen. However, as women approach menopause and estrogen levels decline, this protective fat distribution pattern shifts, leading to more abdominal fat accumulation. This transition contributes to the increased risk of **metabolic syndrome**, **type 2 diabetes**, and **cardiovascular disease** that many women experience during menopause.

For men, **testosterone** is the key hormone that influences muscle mass and fat storage. Testosterone helps promote the development of lean muscle tissue, which is more metabolically active than fat, meaning it burns more calories even at rest. However, as men age, testosterone levels naturally decline, leading to a reduction in muscle mass and an increase in body fat, particularly in the abdominal area. This **abdominal fat**, or **visceral fat**, is metabolically active and can release pro-inflammatory substances, contributing to insulin resistance and other metabolic dysfunctions, as we explored earlier.

The imbalance between estrogen and testosterone can significantly alter how the body stores fat, but these hormones don't act alone. They interact with other hormones, such as **cortisol** and **insulin**, to regulate energy storage, and when these systems become dysregulated, weight gain becomes almost inevitable.

How Hormonal Imbalances Lead to Metabolic Dysfunction

Hormonal imbalances, particularly involving insulin, cortisol, estrogen, and testosterone, can create a perfect storm for weight gain and metabolic dysfunction. Each hormone plays a role in energy balance, and when one is out of sync, it can throw the entire metabolic system off balance.

One of the most common causes of hormonal weight gain is **insulin resistance**, as discussed in Chapter 9.1. When cells become resistant to insulin, blood sugar levels rise, and the body responds by storing more fat, especially in the abdominal area. This leads to **increased fat mass** and makes weight loss extremely challenging, even with diet and exercise interventions.

Cortisol, often referred to as the stress hormone, also plays a major role in weight gain. Chronic stress leads to elevated cortisol levels, which in turn promotes fat storage, particularly in the abdomen. Cortisol also increases appetite and cravings for high-sugar, high-fat foods, leading to **stress eating**. This combination of increased appetite, altered fat distribution, and elevated blood sugar makes it difficult to maintain a healthy weight. In fact, the presence of excess abdominal fat itself can raise cortisol levels, creating a vicious cycle that further promotes weight gain.

Another factor in hormonal weight gain is the **thyroid**, which we've already discussed in Chapter 9.2. The thyroid regulates metabolism, and when it's underactive (hypothyroidism), it slows down the body's ability to burn calories. This reduction in metabolic rate makes it easy to gain weight, even when caloric intake hasn't increased significantly.

In women, **estrogen dominance**—a condition in which estrogen levels are too high relative to progesterone—can lead to weight gain, particularly in the hips, thighs, and abdomen. This imbalance can also increase the risk of **insulin resistance**, further complicating metabolic function. Estrogen dominance is often seen in women with polycystic ovary syndrome (PCOS), a condition that also leads to insulin resistance and weight gain.

In men, low **testosterone** levels can reduce muscle mass, which in turn lowers the metabolic rate, making it easier to gain weight. Low testosterone is also associated with increased fat storage, particularly visceral fat, which is more harmful to metabolic health than subcutaneous fat.

Together, these hormonal imbalances make weight management difficult and increase the risk of developing chronic conditions such as **obesity**, **type 2 diabetes**, and **cardiovascular disease**.

Rebalancing Hormones to Improve Weight Management

Restoring hormonal balance is key to managing weight effectively and preventing the development of metabolic disorders. While medication and hormone therapy are sometimes necessary, many people can achieve significant improvements in their hormonal balance through lifestyle changes.

One of the most effective ways to balance hormones is through **dietary adjustments**. Eating a diet rich in **whole foods** and avoiding processed foods that spike blood sugar and insulin is critical. As we've explored in earlier chapters, balancing macronutrients—particularly by including healthy fats and protein in each meal—can help stabilize blood sugar and insulin levels. Additionally, certain foods can support hormone balance. For example, **flaxseeds** contain **phytoestrogens**, which can help modulate estrogen levels, while **cruciferous vegetables** like broccoli and kale contain compounds that support estrogen metabolism.

In addition to a healthy diet, **regular exercise** plays a critical role in rebalancing hormones. Resistance training, in particular, can help boost testosterone levels in men, promoting muscle growth and improving metabolic rate. For both men and women, incorporating a combination of strength training and cardiovascular exercise can improve insulin sensitivity, reduce cortisol levels, and support overall hormone balance.

Stress management is also essential. As we've discussed in previous chapters, chronic stress raises cortisol levels, which contributes to weight gain. Practicing **mindfulness**, engaging in relaxation techniques, and ensuring sufficient **sleep** can help reduce cortisol levels and support healthy hormonal function. Lack of sleep is one of the most overlooked factors in hormonal imbalances, as insufficient sleep can elevate cortisol, increase ghrelin (the hunger hormone), and decrease leptin (the satiety hormone), leading to increased appetite and weight gain.

Intermittent fasting, as mentioned in Chapter 2.4, can also help rebalance hormones. By providing the body with periods of fasting, insulin levels remain low, and the body is able to burn fat more efficiently. This approach can help reduce insulin resistance and support the balance of other hormones that regulate metabolism.

For individuals experiencing significant hormone imbalances, it's important to **work with a healthcare provider** to get appropriate testing and treatment. Hormone levels can be measured through blood tests, and healthcare providers can recommend targeted interventions, such as hormone replacement therapy, if necessary.

9.4 Cortisol and Its Impact on Metabolic Health

Cortisol, commonly known as the **stress hormone**, is crucial for regulating a wide range of bodily functions, including metabolism, immune response, and energy production.

However, when cortisol levels remain elevated for extended periods due to chronic stress, they can wreak havoc on metabolic health. In this section, we will explore how chronic stress elevates cortisol levels, the long-term effects of high cortisol on the body, and techniques to lower cortisol and improve overall health.

How Chronic Stress Elevates Cortisol Levels

Cortisol is produced by the adrenal glands as part of the body's **fight-or-flight response** to stress. When faced with a stressful situation, the hypothalamus signals the pituitary gland to release **adrenocorticotropic hormone (ACTH)**, which in turn stimulates the adrenal glands to produce cortisol. This hormone helps the body respond to stress by increasing blood sugar levels, suppressing the immune system, and diverting energy to essential functions like muscle contraction and alertness.

In short bursts, cortisol is beneficial, providing the energy and focus needed to handle stressful situations. However, when the body experiences **chronic stress**, cortisol levels remain elevated, disrupting the delicate balance of hormones that regulate metabolism. Over time, this leads to metabolic dysfunction, weight gain, and other health issues.

One of cortisol's main roles during stress is to **increase blood sugar levels** by stimulating the liver to release stored glucose. This is meant to provide the body with a quick source of energy. However, when stress is prolonged, and cortisol remains elevated, blood sugar levels can become persistently high. This, in turn, leads to **insulin resistance**, as discussed earlier in Chapter 9.1. When cells become resistant to insulin, the body struggles to regulate blood sugar effectively, increasing the risk of type 2 diabetes and metabolic syndrome.

Cortisol also has a direct impact on **fat storage**. Under chronic stress, the body tends to store more fat, particularly in the abdominal area. This type of fat, known as **visceral fat**, is especially harmful as it surrounds vital organs and is linked to an increased risk of cardiovascular disease and inflammation. Elevated cortisol levels prompt the body to prioritize fat storage as a survival mechanism, making it difficult to lose weight, even with a healthy diet and regular exercise.

Beyond its impact on blood sugar and fat storage, cortisol affects **appetite** and **cravings**. When cortisol levels are high, the body often craves high-calorie, high-sugar foods as a way to replenish energy quickly. This can lead to overeating and **stress eating**, further contributing to weight gain and metabolic dysfunction. These cravings are part of a feedback loop: stress elevates cortisol, which increases cravings for unhealthy foods, and consuming these foods leads to weight gain and more stress.

The Long-Term Effects of High Cortisol on the Body

Prolonged elevation of cortisol levels can have numerous negative effects on the body, extending beyond metabolism. One of the most significant consequences of chronic high cortisol is its role in **promoting inflammation**. While cortisol is anti-inflammatory in short bursts, chronic stress causes the immune system to become dysregulated, leading to a state of persistent, low-grade inflammation. This inflammation contributes to the development of **chronic diseases**, including cardiovascular disease, type 2 diabetes, and autoimmune disorders.

Chronic stress and high cortisol levels also impact the **digestive system**. Elevated cortisol diverts blood flow away from the digestive tract, impairing digestion and nutrient absorption. Over time, this can lead to gastrointestinal issues such as **irritable bowel syndrome (IBS)**, **leaky gut syndrome**, and other digestive disorders. As digestion becomes less efficient, the body's ability to extract nutrients from food declines, contributing to fatigue and further metabolic dysfunction.

Sleep disturbances are another major consequence of chronic high cortisol. Cortisol follows a natural circadian rhythm, with levels peaking in the morning to help wake the body and decreasing throughout the day. However, chronic stress disrupts this pattern, leading to elevated cortisol levels at night. This can make it difficult to fall asleep or stay asleep, resulting in poor sleep quality. As we explored in Chapter 3, sleep is critical for regulating hormones like insulin, ghrelin, and leptin, all of which are important for metabolic health. Poor sleep further elevates cortisol, creating a vicious cycle of stress, poor sleep, and metabolic dysfunction.

Long-term exposure to high cortisol also affects **muscle mass**. Cortisol breaks down muscle tissue to provide the body with energy during periods of stress. Over time, this **muscle wasting** can reduce the body's overall metabolic rate, making it more difficult to maintain a healthy weight. As muscle mass declines, the body burns fewer calories at rest, further contributing to weight gain and metabolic imbalances.

Chronic high cortisol can also have a significant impact on **mental health**, leading to conditions such as **anxiety**, **depression**, and **burnout**. Cortisol affects neurotransmitters like serotonin and dopamine, which regulate mood and emotional well-being. Persistent stress can lead to a depletion of these neurotransmitters, contributing to feelings of anxiety and depression. Additionally, the cognitive effects of chronic stress, such as difficulty concentrating and memory problems, can impair quality of life.

Techniques to Lower Cortisol and Improve Overall Health

Fortunately, there are many effective strategies to lower cortisol levels and improve overall health. One of the most important steps is to manage stress more effectively. While it's impossible to eliminate stress entirely, incorporating stress-reduction techniques into daily life can help keep cortisol levels in check.

Mindfulness meditation is one of the most researched and effective tools for reducing cortisol. As mentioned in Chapter 8.4, mindfulness helps the body shift from a stress response to a state of relaxation by activating the parasympathetic nervous system. This practice can be as simple as focusing on your breath for a few minutes each day, allowing the body to reset and reduce cortisol levels.

Exercise is another powerful way to manage cortisol, but it's important to strike the right balance. While intense, prolonged exercise can temporarily increase cortisol levels, moderate exercise, such as walking, yoga, or swimming, helps to lower cortisol and improve overall metabolic function. Regular physical activity enhances **insulin sensitivity**, reduces stress, and supports hormone balance, making it a key tool in managing both cortisol and weight.

In addition to stress management techniques, **sleep** plays a critical role in regulating cortisol levels. As we explored in earlier chapters, improving sleep hygiene by maintaining a consistent bedtime, avoiding screens before bed, and creating a relaxing sleep environment can help restore the body's natural cortisol rhythm. Getting enough restorative sleep is essential for lowering cortisol and supporting metabolic health.

Nutrition also plays an important role in managing cortisol levels. Eating a balanced diet that includes plenty of vegetables, fruits, lean proteins, and healthy fats can help stabilize blood sugar and reduce stress on the body. Foods rich in **omega-3 fatty acids**, such as salmon and flaxseeds, have anti-inflammatory properties that help regulate cortisol levels. Avoiding **stimulants** like caffeine and sugar, especially in the evening, can prevent cortisol spikes and support better sleep.

Finally, engaging in **social connections** and maintaining strong relationships can help reduce stress and lower cortisol. Studies show that individuals who have strong social support networks tend to have lower cortisol levels and are better able to manage stress. Whether through family, friends, or support groups, staying connected with others provides emotional resilience and helps protect against the harmful effects of chronic stress.

9.5 Balancing Hormones Through Natural Interventions

Balancing hormones naturally is essential for maintaining metabolic health, energy levels, and overall well-being. Many of the hormones responsible for regulating metabolism, fat storage, and energy production can be influenced through lifestyle choices, nutrition, and natural interventions. In this section, we'll explore key nutrients that support hormonal balance, the role of **adaptogens** in regulating hormones, and how **sleep** and **relaxation** help restore hormonal equilibrium.

Nutrients That Support Hormonal Balance

The food you eat plays a critical role in how your body produces and regulates hormones. Certain nutrients are particularly important for maintaining hormonal balance and can be incorporated into your daily diet to support the endocrine system. A focus on whole, nutrient-dense foods ensures that your body has the building blocks it needs to produce and regulate hormones effectively.

One of the most important nutrients for hormonal balance is **omega-3 fatty acids**, which have anti-inflammatory properties that support the regulation of several hormones, including insulin, cortisol, and sex hormones like estrogen and testosterone. Omega-3s can be found in foods like **fatty fish** (salmon, mackerel, sardines), **chia seeds**, **flaxseeds**, and

walnuts. These healthy fats help stabilize blood sugar, reduce inflammation, and improve insulin sensitivity—key factors in managing hormonal health.

Magnesium is another essential nutrient for balancing hormones, especially when it comes to stress management. Magnesium helps regulate cortisol levels, promotes relaxation, and improves sleep quality, all of which are important for hormonal equilibrium. Foods rich in magnesium include **leafy greens** (spinach, kale), **almonds**, **pumpkin seeds**, and **dark chocolate**. A magnesium deficiency is often linked to higher stress levels and poor sleep, which can throw off the balance of hormones like cortisol and melatonin.

Zinc is a critical mineral for the production of sex hormones, including estrogen and testosterone. It also supports the immune system and helps regulate the menstrual cycle in women. Foods like **oysters**, **pumpkin seeds**, **chickpeas**, and **beef** are excellent sources of zinc. A diet lacking in zinc can lead to hormonal imbalances, reduced fertility, and disrupted metabolic function.

B vitamins, particularly **B6**, **B12**, and **folate**, are essential for hormone production and regulation. These vitamins help convert food into energy and play a role in synthesizing neurotransmitters, which are involved in mood regulation and stress responses. B vitamins are found in a variety of foods, including **whole grains**, **eggs**, **leafy greens**, and **legumes**. Ensuring adequate intake of B vitamins can help support adrenal function, improve energy levels, and regulate estrogen and progesterone.

In addition to these nutrients, **fiber** plays a key role in supporting hormonal balance by promoting healthy digestion and aiding in the elimination of excess hormones, particularly estrogen. Soluble fiber, found in foods like **oats**, **apples**, **beans**, and **sweet potatoes**, helps the body detoxify and manage estrogen levels, reducing the risk of estrogen dominance, which is linked to conditions like polycystic ovary syndrome (PCOS) and certain cancers.

The Role of Adaptogens in Hormonal Health

Adaptogens are a unique class of herbs and plants that help the body adapt to stress and restore balance to the endocrine system. They are particularly effective at regulating cortisol levels, which play a major role in stress response and overall hormonal balance. By modulating the body's stress response, adaptogens can help prevent the long-term effects of elevated cortisol, such as insulin resistance, weight gain, and inflammation.

One of the most well-known adaptogens is **ashwagandha**, an herb traditionally used in Ayurvedic medicine. Ashwagandha helps lower cortisol levels, improve thyroid function, and balance sex hormones. Studies have shown that ashwagandha can reduce stress and anxiety, improve energy levels, and support metabolic health. It's particularly beneficial for individuals experiencing **adrenal fatigue**—a condition where the adrenal glands become overworked due to chronic stress, resulting in hormonal imbalances.

Another powerful adaptogen is **rhodiola**, which is known for its ability to combat fatigue, reduce stress, and enhance mental clarity. Rhodiola supports the adrenal glands and helps the body cope with both physical and emotional stress. By balancing cortisol levels, rhodiola can help improve insulin sensitivity and regulate appetite, making it a valuable tool for managing stress-related weight gain.

Maca root is another adaptogen that has gained popularity for its ability to balance sex hormones, particularly estrogen and progesterone. It's often used to support reproductive health, improve fertility, and reduce symptoms of menopause. Maca helps balance the **hypothalamic-pituitary-adrenal (HPA) axis**, which regulates the body's stress response, and can improve energy levels and mood.

Holy basil, also known as **tulsi**, is another adaptogen that helps reduce cortisol levels and promotes relaxation. It has been used for centuries in traditional medicine to support the immune system and balance hormones. Holy basil is particularly beneficial for individuals who experience anxiety and mental fatigue due to high stress levels, as it helps calm the mind and body.

Incorporating adaptogens into your daily routine can help restore hormonal balance by regulating cortisol, supporting adrenal health, and improving the body's resilience to stress. These herbs are typically available as supplements, teas, or powders and can be easily added to smoothies, drinks, or taken in capsule form.

How Sleep and Relaxation Restore Hormonal Equilibrium

Sleep is one of the most important factors for maintaining hormonal balance, yet it is often overlooked in discussions about health and wellness. The body's hormones follow natural cycles that are regulated by the **circadian rhythm**—the body's internal clock that governs sleep-wake cycles, energy levels, and hormone production. When sleep is disrupted, these hormonal cycles become imbalanced, leading to metabolic dysfunction, weight gain, and increased stress.

As we discussed in Chapter 3, **melatonin**, the hormone responsible for regulating sleep, plays a key role in this process. Melatonin levels rise in the evening, helping to induce sleep, and decrease in the morning to signal wakefulness. However, chronic stress, poor sleep hygiene, and exposure to artificial light can disrupt melatonin production, making it difficult to fall asleep or stay asleep. Without adequate sleep, cortisol levels remain elevated, further disrupting the balance of other hormones like insulin, ghrelin, and leptin, which regulate appetite and metabolism.

To restore hormonal equilibrium, it's crucial to prioritize **quality sleep**. Establishing a consistent sleep routine—going to bed and waking up at the same time each day—helps regulate the circadian rhythm and improve the production of key hormones. Limiting exposure to blue light from screens in the evening, creating a dark, quiet sleep environment, and avoiding stimulants like caffeine before bed can all support better sleep quality.

Relaxation techniques such as **meditation, deep breathing**, and **yoga** can also play a significant role in restoring hormonal balance. These practices activate the **parasympathetic nervous system**, which promotes relaxation and reduces cortisol levels. As cortisol levels drop, the body is better able to regulate other hormones, improving overall metabolic health and well-being.

Additionally, ensuring adequate relaxation during the day—by taking breaks, spending time in nature, or engaging in activities you enjoy—can help keep stress levels in check and prevent cortisol from remaining elevated. Over time, these small changes can have a profound impact on hormone regulation, improving both physical and mental health.

Chapter 10: Immune Function and Metabolic Health

The immune system and metabolic health are deeply interconnected, influencing how the body responds to both internal and external threats. Chronic inflammation, often driven by poor diet, stress, and environmental toxins, can disrupt metabolic processes and lead to conditions such as insulin resistance, obesity, and cardiovascular disease. On the other hand, a well-functioning metabolism supports a healthy immune response, allowing the body to effectively fight infections and prevent illness.

Inflammation, which is a natural immune response, can become problematic when it persists over time. This chronic state of inflammation is closely tied to metabolic dysfunction and contributes to the development of many chronic diseases. The gut microbiome also plays a crucial role in regulating immune responses and metabolic health, highlighting the importance of gut health for overall well-being.

In this chapter, we will explore how the immune system and metabolism are linked, focusing on the role of chronic inflammation, immune-related metabolic disorders, and strategies for enhancing immune function through improved metabolic health. We will also look at how lifestyle factors, such as diet, exercise, and stress management, can help reduce inflammation and support a stronger immune system.

10.1 The Link Between Inflammation and Metabolism

Inflammation is a natural, protective response designed to help the body recover from injury or fight off infection. But what happens when this defense mechanism doesn't turn off? Chronic inflammation can significantly disrupt metabolic function, leading to a cascade of health issues. To fully understand how **chronic inflammation** impacts metabolism, we need to explore the pathways that connect immune responses with energy regulation.

How Chronic Inflammation Disrupts Metabolic Function

At the heart of chronic inflammation is the body's immune system, which, when activated for prolonged periods, sends constant signals to defend itself against perceived threats. This ongoing response can interfere with essential cellular processes, including **insulin sensitivity**, energy production, and fat storage.

One of the first systems to feel the effects of chronic inflammation is **insulin signaling**. Inflammation disrupts the ability of cells to respond to insulin, a hormone critical for regulating blood sugar levels. **Cytokines**, which are molecules released by immune cells during inflammation, interfere with insulin receptors on cells, making them less effective at absorbing glucose. This leads to **insulin resistance**, where more insulin is required to lower blood sugar levels, which in turn leads to increased insulin production. Over time, this state not only heightens the risk of developing **type 2 diabetes**, but it also triggers the body to store more fat, particularly around the abdomen.

This is where the cycle becomes self-reinforcing. **Visceral fat**, the type that accumulates around internal organs, isn't just passive tissue; it actively contributes to inflammation by releasing its own inflammatory molecules, further worsening metabolic dysfunction. This kind of fat is strongly linked to heart disease, metabolic syndrome, and other chronic conditions.

The impact of chronic inflammation extends beyond insulin and fat storage. It also affects **mitochondria**, the energy producers of the cell. Inflammatory molecules damage mitochondrial function, reducing the cell's ability to produce **adenosine triphosphate (ATP)**, the body's primary energy currency. When cells can't produce enough energy, the result is **chronic fatigue**, sluggishness, and an overall slower metabolism. This diminished capacity to generate energy directly impairs the body's ability to burn calories efficiently, making weight loss and energy maintenance difficult.

This brings us to a broader question: if inflammation can disrupt so many metabolic processes, what are the underlying triggers? To answer this, we need to look at some of the most common dietary and environmental factors that promote inflammation.

Common Dietary and Environmental Triggers

Many modern lifestyle factors contribute to chronic inflammation. One of the most prevalent is the **Western diet**, characterized by its reliance on **processed foods**, refined carbohydrates, and unhealthy fats. These foods, while convenient, are filled with **pro-inflammatory ingredients**, such as **trans fats** and **excess sugar**. They cause spikes in blood sugar levels and create oxidative stress, both of which trigger inflammatory pathways.

Consider a typical fast-food meal. The combination of refined carbohydrates from the bun, unhealthy fats from fried components, and sugar from sodas leads to a sharp increase in blood sugar. Over time, this pattern of eating primes the body for **insulin resistance** and elevates levels of inflammatory cytokines.

But it's not just diet. **Environmental toxins** also play a significant role in chronic inflammation. Exposure to pollutants, chemicals in cleaning products, and pesticides in non-organic foods introduces harmful substances into the body, where they disrupt cellular function. These toxins are often absorbed and stored in fat tissue, which can further contribute to inflammation. The more toxic buildup the body has to manage, the more prolonged the inflammatory response becomes.

Chronic stress and **sleep deprivation** further amplify inflammation. As we discussed earlier in Chapter 9, stress elevates **cortisol**, a hormone that, when chronically elevated, leads to increased fat storage and inflammation. **Lack of sleep** compounds the issue by preventing the body from performing its nightly repair functions, leaving the immune system in a constant state of alert.

What does all this mean for our metabolic health? Simply put, chronic exposure to inflammatory triggers sets the stage for a slow, steady decline in metabolic function, making it harder for the body to regulate weight, energy, and blood sugar.

Anti-Inflammatory Practices to Restore Balance

Given how profoundly inflammation affects metabolism, the key to restoring balance lies in adopting **anti-inflammatory practices**. One of the most impactful steps is to shift toward an **anti-inflammatory diet**, prioritizing whole, nutrient-dense foods that actively reduce inflammation.

Omega-3 fatty acids are among the most powerful dietary tools for fighting inflammation. Found in foods like **salmon**, **flaxseeds**, and **chia seeds**, omega-3s help reduce the production of inflammatory cytokines. Studies consistently show that individuals who consume omega-3s regularly have lower levels of **C-reactive protein (CRP)**, a marker of inflammation, and improved insulin sensitivity.

Alongside omega-3s, **antioxidants** play a critical role in reducing oxidative stress, which contributes to inflammation. Foods rich in antioxidants, such as **berries, green tea, leafy greens**, and **nuts**, help neutralize free radicals—unstable molecules that damage cells and trigger inflammation. In particular, **polyphenols** in foods like olive oil and turmeric have been shown to protect against oxidative damage while supporting the body's anti-inflammatory pathways.

But reducing inflammation through diet isn't just about what you add—it's also about what you remove. Avoiding processed foods, refined sugars, and trans fats is essential for lowering inflammatory markers. These foods not only disrupt insulin levels but also increase levels of **pro-inflammatory eicosanoids**, which further exacerbate metabolic dysfunction.

Beyond dietary changes, **physical activity** is another effective way to manage inflammation. Regular moderate exercise has been shown to lower inflammatory markers and improve metabolic health by enhancing **insulin sensitivity** and reducing visceral fat. Activities like walking, cycling, and strength training provide a protective effect against the damaging consequences of chronic inflammation.

Managing **stress** is essential for controlling inflammation. Chronic stress, as discussed in Chapter 9.4, keeps cortisol elevated and perpetuates the inflammatory cycle. Incorporating **mindfulness practices**, such as meditation, yoga, or even deep breathing exercises, can help reduce cortisol levels and shift the body out of its constant state of alert.

Finally, reducing exposure to **environmental toxins** is an often overlooked but crucial component of lowering inflammation. By choosing **organic produce**, using **natural cleaning products**, and limiting exposure to harmful chemicals in everyday items, you can lessen the toxic load your body has to manage. Supporting your body's detoxification processes—through adequate hydration, as mentioned in Chapter 2, and consuming fiber-rich foods—further aids in this effort.

The intricate link between inflammation and metabolism is a powerful reminder of how interconnected our systems truly are. Chronic inflammation not only impairs insulin sensitivity and energy production but also leads to long-term metabolic dysfunction. By adopting anti-inflammatory practices through diet, lifestyle changes, and stress management, you can help restore balance to both your immune system and your metabolism, paving the way for improved energy, weight regulation, and overall health.

10.2 Immune Function's Role in Energy Production

The immune system, typically recognized for its role in defending the body against infections, also plays a significant role in **energy production** at the cellular level. This connection between immune function and metabolism is vital for maintaining overall health and ensuring that the body can effectively respond to both internal and external stressors. When the immune system is functioning properly, it supports cellular health and metabolic efficiency. However, an overactive or compromised immune response can lead to **metabolic inefficiency**, fatigue, and a range of chronic conditions.

How the Immune System Affects Cellular Health

At the core of energy production is the cell, and more specifically, the **mitochondria**—the powerhouse of the cell responsible for producing **adenosine triphosphate (ATP)**, the energy currency used by the body for nearly all biological processes. The immune system interacts closely with mitochondrial function, ensuring that cells can meet energy demands during periods of stress, infection, or injury.

When the body is under stress, whether from a pathogen or physical injury, the immune system launches an inflammatory response to contain the threat. This process is necessary for healing, but it also diverts resources, including energy, to the immune system. **Cytokines**, small proteins released by immune cells, communicate with mitochondria, influencing how much energy the cell produces. During acute inflammation, energy production increases to fuel the immune system's response, but when inflammation becomes chronic, this energy demand remains high, eventually overwhelming the body's ability to maintain efficient energy production.

In cases of **chronic inflammation**, immune cells produce a constant flow of inflammatory signals, such as **interleukin-6 (IL-6)** and **tumor necrosis factor-alpha (TNF-α)**. These cytokines can impair mitochondrial function, reducing their ability to produce ATP efficiently. This leads to a condition known as **mitochondrial dysfunction**, where cells produce less energy than needed, resulting in **fatigue** and sluggish metabolic processes. Mitochondrial dysfunction also accelerates the breakdown of muscle tissue, further decreasing energy production and leading to muscle weakness and metabolic slowdown.

What's more, an overactive immune response can cause oxidative stress—an imbalance between free radicals and antioxidants in the body. This oxidative stress damages mitochondria, reducing their capacity to produce energy, and leading to **cellular damage**. Over time, this damage contributes to the development of **insulin resistance**, type 2 diabetes, and other metabolic disorders.

The intricate balance between immune function and energy production highlights why chronic inflammation can leave people feeling fatigued and depleted, even in the absence of infection. The immune system's need for energy diverts resources from other cellular functions, impacting metabolic efficiency and leading to a reduction in the body's overall energy output.

Immune Responses and Metabolic Efficiency

When immune function is compromised or constantly active due to chronic inflammation, the body's ability to manage energy efficiently is significantly impaired. Normally, when the immune system is at rest, the body directs energy toward essential metabolic functions like digestion, muscle repair, and maintaining body temperature. However, when the immune system is constantly engaged in fighting off perceived threats, this energy is redirected to support immune responses, leaving fewer resources available for other critical processes.

A key example of this is seen during acute infections. During an infection, the body temporarily shifts its energy priorities. For instance, when dealing with a bacterial infection, energy is diverted away from fat burning or muscle building and instead used to fuel immune cells that need to proliferate quickly to eliminate the threat. This is a **short-term trade-off** that benefits survival. However, when the immune system is constantly in a state of low-grade activation, as is the case with chronic inflammation, this energy diversion becomes a long-term issue, leading to **metabolic inefficiency**.

The body's immune responses can also affect **blood sugar regulation**. When inflammatory cytokines are released, they signal the liver to release **glucose** into the bloodstream as part of the body's fight-or-flight response. This glucose provides quick energy to immune cells that need it. However, if this process happens too frequently, it can contribute to **insulin resistance**, making it more difficult for the body to manage blood sugar levels. Over time, this dysregulation leads to a host of metabolic problems, including **type 2 diabetes** and **obesity**.

Immune-mediated energy inefficiency is further compounded by **muscle loss** during chronic inflammation. When the body is in a prolonged inflammatory state, the immune system can cause muscle catabolism, where proteins in muscle tissue are broken down to provide energy for immune cells. This loss of muscle mass decreases the body's overall metabolic rate, as muscle tissue is more metabolically active than fat. This creates a feedback loop where inflammation promotes muscle loss, leading to lower energy production and a slower metabolism.

Strengthening Immune Function to Improve Energy Levels

Given the close relationship between the immune system and energy production, improving immune health is essential for boosting metabolic efficiency and overall vitality. Strengthening immune function can help restore energy balance and support more efficient metabolism.

Diet plays a crucial role in supporting both immune function and energy production. As discussed in Chapter 9.5, consuming foods rich in **antioxidants, omega-3 fatty acids**, and **micronutrients** helps reduce chronic inflammation and protect against mitochondrial damage. Omega-3s, found in fatty fish like salmon, as well as flaxseeds and walnuts, help regulate immune responses and prevent excessive cytokine production. **Antioxidants**, found in berries, leafy greens, and green tea, neutralize free radicals and reduce oxidative stress, protecting mitochondria from damage.

Incorporating **probiotic-rich foods** like yogurt, kefir, and fermented vegetables can also support immune function by promoting a healthy gut microbiome, which plays a key role in regulating inflammation and immune responses. A balanced gut microbiome helps prevent the overproduction of inflammatory cytokines and ensures that the immune system responds appropriately to threats without overreacting.

Regular **physical activity** is another powerful way to boost immune function and improve energy levels. Moderate-intensity exercise, such as walking, swimming, or yoga, has been shown to lower inflammation and enhance mitochondrial function, improving both energy production and metabolic health. Exercise increases blood flow and oxygen delivery to cells, supporting ATP production and promoting cellular repair.

Adequate **sleep** is perhaps one of the most important factors for maintaining a healthy immune system and supporting energy production. As discussed in Chapter 3, sleep is critical for immune regulation, as the body uses this time to repair damaged tissues and modulate immune responses. Lack of sleep can increase inflammation, disrupt glucose metabolism, and lead to mitochondrial dysfunction. Ensuring quality sleep by maintaining a consistent sleep schedule, reducing screen time before bed, and creating a relaxing sleep environment is crucial for restoring immune balance and metabolic efficiency.

Stress management is essential for maintaining immune health. Chronic stress elevates cortisol levels, which, as we've seen in previous chapters, can promote inflammation and impair mitochondrial function. Incorporating **mindfulness practices**, such as meditation, deep breathing, and relaxation techniques, can help reduce stress and support both immune function and energy production.

Understanding the intricate relationship between the immune system and energy production underscores the importance of maintaining a balanced immune response for optimal metabolic health. By strengthening immune function through proper nutrition, regular exercise, quality sleep, and stress management, the body can produce energy more efficiently, reduce inflammation, and promote overall well-being. The more efficiently your immune system functions, the better equipped your body is to manage energy and maintain metabolic balance, ensuring sustained energy levels and improved health outcomes.

10.3 Autoimmunity and Metabolic Dysfunction

Autoimmune conditions occur when the body's immune system mistakenly attacks its own healthy cells, mistaking them for foreign invaders. This improper immune response can have profound effects on metabolic health, leading to **metabolic dysfunction**, weight fluctuations, and chronic fatigue. Understanding the link between **autoimmunity** and metabolism is essential for managing both autoimmune conditions and the metabolic issues they cause.

The Connection Between Autoimmune Conditions and Metabolism

Autoimmune diseases, such as **Hashimoto's thyroiditis, rheumatoid arthritis, type 1 diabetes**, and **lupus**, are characterized by persistent inflammation. This chronic inflammation results from the immune system's ongoing attack on the body's tissues. In autoimmune conditions, the immune response not only damages specific organs but also disrupts metabolic processes.

In **Hashimoto's thyroiditis**, for example, the immune system attacks the thyroid gland, impairing its ability to produce thyroid hormones. The thyroid is responsible for regulating metabolism, so when its function is compromised, the result is **hypothyroidism**, where the body's metabolic rate slows down. This leads to **weight gain, fatigue, insulin resistance**, and difficulty regulating body temperature. Similarly, **type 1 diabetes** results from the immune system targeting and destroying the insulin-producing cells in the pancreas. Without insulin, glucose cannot be absorbed into cells efficiently, causing blood sugar levels to spike and leading to serious metabolic imbalances.

What's crucial to note is that the inflammation triggered by autoimmune conditions not only affects the specific organ under attack but also has broader metabolic consequences. **Systemic inflammation**—a hallmark of autoimmune diseases—disrupts **insulin signaling**, impairs mitochondrial function, and promotes **fat storage**, particularly around the abdomen. These effects make it harder to maintain stable blood sugar levels and manage body weight, even with a healthy diet and regular exercise.

Moreover, chronic inflammation contributes to **mitochondrial dysfunction**, reducing the body's ability to produce energy efficiently. This leads to **chronic fatigue**, a common symptom in many autoimmune conditions, where individuals feel persistently exhausted despite adequate rest. This fatigue is more than just tiredness; it's a sign that the body's metabolic machinery is not functioning optimally due to the immune system's constant overactivity.

Recognizing Early Signs of Autoimmunity

Early detection of autoimmune conditions is key to managing both the immune response and the metabolic issues that arise as a result. However, autoimmune diseases often present with vague or nonspecific symptoms, making diagnosis difficult in the early stages. Common early signs include **unexplained weight changes, persistent fatigue, joint pain**, and **digestive issues**.

For example, in **Hashimoto's thyroiditis**, individuals may notice **unexplained weight gain, constipation, dry skin**, and **feeling cold**, all of which are related to a slowing metabolism. In contrast, someone with **type 1 diabetes** might experience **frequent urination, excessive thirst**, and **unintended weight loss** as a result of the body's inability to manage blood sugar effectively.

Autoimmune conditions also often cause **brain fog**—a feeling of mental cloudiness or difficulty concentrating—which is closely tied to the metabolic disruptions caused by inflammation. As inflammation interferes with insulin signaling and mitochondrial function, the brain's ability to use glucose for energy becomes impaired, leading to cognitive issues.

Another sign of autoimmunity is **persistent inflammation** that doesn't seem to have an obvious cause, such as ongoing joint pain or swelling in the absence of injury. These symptoms are the result of the immune system attacking healthy tissues, causing chronic pain and discomfort. Recognizing these early signs and seeking medical evaluation can help in diagnosing autoimmune conditions before they cause further metabolic damage.

Dietary and Lifestyle Strategies for Autoimmune Conditions

Managing autoimmune conditions requires a comprehensive approach that addresses both the immune system's overactivity and the resulting metabolic dysfunction. One of the most effective ways to manage autoimmune symptoms and improve metabolic health is through **dietary changes** that reduce inflammation and support immune balance.

The **anti-inflammatory diet**, discussed in earlier chapters, is especially beneficial for individuals with autoimmune conditions. This diet emphasizes whole foods rich in **omega-3 fatty acids**, **antioxidants**, and **fiber**, all of which help lower inflammation. Foods like **salmon, chia seeds, leafy greens, berries**, and **cruciferous vegetables** can reduce the production of inflammatory cytokines and support overall immune health.

In addition to anti-inflammatory foods, certain **nutritional interventions** can specifically benefit individuals with autoimmune conditions. For example, people with **Hashimoto's thyroiditis** often benefit from ensuring adequate intake of **selenium** and **zinc**, two minerals that support thyroid function and help regulate the immune response. Brazil nuts are a rich source of selenium, while zinc can be found in foods like **pumpkin seeds** and **beef**.

In individuals with **celiac disease**, an autoimmune condition triggered by gluten, a **strict gluten-free diet** is essential for reducing inflammation and preventing further damage to the small intestine. Even trace amounts of gluten can provoke an immune response, so eliminating gluten entirely is necessary to improve both immune function and metabolic health.

Gut health is another critical area for managing autoimmunity and metabolic function. Since a significant portion of the immune system is housed in the gut, maintaining a healthy gut microbiome is essential for regulating immune responses. **Probiotics**, found in fermented foods like **yogurt, sauerkraut**, and **kimchi**, support a balanced microbiome and help reduce inflammation. Consuming foods rich in **prebiotics**, such as garlic, onions, and asparagus, can also nourish beneficial gut bacteria.

Beyond diet, **stress management** plays a crucial role in controlling autoimmune flare-ups and improving metabolic function. Chronic stress exacerbates inflammation and can trigger autoimmune symptoms by elevating cortisol levels, which, in turn, leads to insulin resistance and metabolic disruption. Practices like **meditation, deep breathing**, and **yoga** can help reduce stress and promote relaxation, calming the immune system.

Regular **exercise** is another important lifestyle factor for managing autoimmunity. While intense exercise can sometimes trigger inflammation, moderate activities like **walking, swimming**, or **gentle yoga** have been shown to lower inflammatory markers and support metabolic health. Exercise also helps reduce fatigue, improve mood, and regulate blood sugar, all of which are critical for individuals with autoimmune conditions.

Lastly, **sleep** is essential for managing both immune function and metabolism. As discussed in Chapter 3, quality sleep allows the body to repair tissues, regulate immune responses, and restore energy levels. Sleep deprivation, on the other hand, increases inflammation and disrupts metabolic processes. Ensuring consistent, restful sleep can help prevent autoimmune flare-ups and support long-term health.

Managing autoimmune conditions requires addressing both the immune system's overactivity and the resulting metabolic dysfunction. By recognizing the early signs of autoimmunity, adopting an anti-inflammatory diet, supporting gut health, and incorporating stress management and regular exercise, individuals with autoimmune conditions can reduce inflammation, improve energy levels, and maintain better metabolic health. Balancing the immune system is not only crucial for managing autoimmune symptoms but also for restoring metabolic equilibrium and preventing long-term health complications.

10.4 Metabolic Health for Disease Prevention

Metabolism is at the core of how our body functions daily, influencing not only our energy levels but also our overall health and susceptibility to chronic illnesses. From insulin regulation to inflammation control, metabolism plays a crucial role in disease prevention. When it functions optimally, it helps us maintain balance, fight infections, and keep our systems running smoothly. On the other hand, a sluggish or impaired metabolism can increase the risk of diseases like type 2 diabetes, cardiovascular disease, and autoimmune disorders. Understanding how **metabolic health** contributes to disease prevention and learning the steps to support it are key to maintaining long-term wellness.

The Role of Metabolism in Preventing Illness

To fully grasp the role of metabolism in disease prevention, it's important to think beyond its function as a mere calorie-burning machine. Metabolism manages how effectively our body converts food into energy, regulates hormone levels, controls inflammation, and keeps blood sugar stable—all crucial factors for avoiding chronic diseases. When metabolism is running efficiently, it supports the body's ability to fight off illness and keep inflammation at bay. But what happens when metabolic function falters?

One of the most common ways metabolism contributes to illness is through **insulin resistance**. As we discussed in earlier chapters, insulin is the hormone that helps cells absorb glucose from the bloodstream. When cells become resistant to insulin, the body produces more of it, resulting in **hyperinsulinemia** (excess insulin in the blood). Over time, this leads to elevated blood sugar levels, which can damage blood vessels, increase inflammation, and contribute to fat storage, particularly **visceral fat**. This type of fat surrounds internal organs and is associated with a higher risk of heart disease, stroke, and metabolic syndrome.

The presence of chronic inflammation is another key player in the breakdown of metabolic health. Inflammation, when it's a temporary response to injury or infection, is part of the body's defense system. But **chronic inflammation**—a low-level, persistent state of immune activation—can disrupt metabolic processes and lead to diseases. Inflammation impairs the body's ability to regulate insulin, damages mitochondria (the powerhouses of the cell), and slows down energy production. Over time, this can create a domino effect: fatigue sets in, weight gain becomes harder to control, and metabolic efficiency declines.

But there's more at stake. The **mitochondria** are essential for producing the energy (in the form of ATP) that our cells need to function. When inflammation impairs mitochondrial function, cells lose their ability to efficiently convert food into usable energy. This decline in energy production not only contributes to feelings of fatigue but also makes it harder for the body to recover from stress or illness. In this state, the immune system is compromised, making it harder to fight infections and increasing the risk of developing chronic diseases.

Ultimately, metabolic health serves as a protective barrier against illness. When it functions properly, it stabilizes blood sugar, maintains energy levels, and regulates the body's response to inflammation. This balance is key for preventing many common chronic diseases.

Optimizing Metabolism for Stronger Defenses

Optimizing metabolism is a powerful way to strengthen the body's natural defenses and protect against disease. When metabolism is functioning at its best, it regulates hormones, keeps energy production efficient, and maintains a healthy balance of **insulin sensitivity** and **inflammatory control**. By making targeted changes to your lifestyle, you can enhance your metabolic health and, in turn, bolster your body's ability to prevent illness.

One of the most critical factors in metabolic health is **insulin sensitivity**. When cells are sensitive to insulin, they can absorb glucose effectively, which helps regulate blood sugar levels and reduce the risk of insulin resistance. Improving insulin sensitivity can be achieved through several strategies, including regular physical activity, a balanced diet, and managing stress levels. As we explored in previous chapters, **physical exercise** is particularly important because it helps muscle cells become more responsive to insulin, allowing them to take in glucose without needing as much insulin. This not only helps manage blood sugar but also lowers inflammation, creating a healthier internal environment.

Hormonal balance is equally important for optimizing metabolism. Hormones such as **cortisol, thyroid hormones**, and **insulin** govern many of the body's key metabolic functions, including how we manage energy and store fat. When these hormones are out of balance—often due to chronic stress, poor sleep, or an unhealthy diet—metabolic processes slow down, and the immune system becomes less efficient. Chronic stress, in particular, can lead to elevated cortisol levels, which promote fat storage around the abdomen and contribute to **insulin resistance**. Managing stress through relaxation techniques, such as **meditation** or **yoga**, and ensuring adequate sleep are essential for keeping hormones in check and supporting overall metabolic health.

Mitochondrial health is another vital area to consider. Mitochondria are responsible for producing the energy that powers nearly every function in the body. When mitochondrial function declines—due to factors like poor diet, oxidative stress, or inflammation—cells become less efficient at converting nutrients into energy, leading to fatigue, weight gain, and increased susceptibility to disease. To support mitochondrial function, it's important to focus on nutrition. Consuming a diet rich in **antioxidants** helps neutralize free radicals, which can damage mitochondria. Foods like berries, leafy greens, and nuts are excellent sources of antioxidants that support cellular health.

Another key aspect of optimizing metabolism is maintaining a **balanced diet** that promotes insulin sensitivity and reduces inflammation. Foods rich in **omega-3 fatty acids**, such as fatty fish, flaxseeds, and walnuts, are well-known for their anti-inflammatory properties. They help reduce the production of inflammatory cytokines, which can disrupt insulin signaling and promote fat storage. Similarly, incorporating **fiber-rich foods** like whole grains, legumes, and vegetables helps regulate blood sugar and supports a healthy gut microbiome, which plays a role in both immune function and metabolic health.

Physical activity is one of the most effective ways to improve metabolic efficiency. Regular exercise not only enhances **insulin sensitivity** but also promotes **mitochondrial biogenesis**, the process by which the body creates new mitochondria. This increases the body's ability to produce energy and improves overall metabolic function. Even moderate-intensity activities like walking, swimming, or resistance training can have profound effects on both metabolic and immune health.

Steps to Support Immunity Through Metabolic Health

To fully support both metabolic health and immune function, a holistic approach is needed. Strengthening your metabolism can enhance your body's defenses and reduce the risk of developing chronic diseases. Here are some key steps to integrate into your daily routine:

First, focus on maintaining a **balanced, nutrient-dense diet**. As mentioned earlier, whole foods that are rich in **antioxidants**, **omega-3s**, and **fiber** play an essential role in reducing inflammation and supporting metabolic processes. Avoid processed foods and refined sugars, as they can lead to blood sugar spikes, insulin resistance, and inflammation, all of which weaken the immune system.

Incorporating regular **physical activity** is another vital step. Exercise improves insulin sensitivity and enhances mitochondrial function, both of which are crucial for maintaining energy levels and regulating blood sugar. A mix of aerobic exercise, such as brisk walking or swimming, combined with resistance training, helps improve overall metabolic function while reducing fat stores that contribute to inflammation.

Stress management is equally important. Chronic stress disrupts hormonal balance, leading to elevated cortisol levels, which in turn promote insulin resistance and fat accumulation. Practices like **deep breathing**, **meditation**, and **progressive muscle relaxation** can help lower cortisol and improve both metabolic and immune health.

Adequate **sleep** is critical for maintaining metabolic balance and immune function. Poor sleep impairs insulin sensitivity, increases inflammation, and disrupts hormone levels. By creating a consistent sleep routine and ensuring 7-9 hours of restful sleep each night, you can support both your metabolism and your body's natural defenses.

Finally, ensure you are well **hydrated** and supporting your body's natural detoxification processes. Drinking enough water helps flush toxins from the body, aids in digestion, and supports cellular function. Hydration also plays a role in maintaining the body's temperature and improving nutrient absorption, which are important for both metabolic efficiency and immune strength.

By focusing on metabolic health, you lay the foundation for a body that not only has the energy to thrive but also possesses the defenses needed to fend off chronic diseases. Through a combination of balanced nutrition, regular exercise, stress management, and quality sleep, you can optimize metabolism and enhance your overall well-being. When metabolism works efficiently, your body can more effectively regulate blood sugar, control inflammation, and support immune function, ultimately protecting you from illness and promoting a healthier, more resilient life.

10.5 The Microbiome's Role in Immune Health

In recent years, the **gut microbiome** has emerged as a central factor influencing both metabolic and immune health. This complex ecosystem of bacteria, viruses, and fungi that live in the digestive tract plays a pivotal role in regulating digestion, nutrient absorption, and the body's immune responses. The health of the gut microbiome is directly linked to the body's ability to manage inflammation, regulate metabolism, and fend off illness. In this section, we will explore how the gut microbiome influences immune function, the dietary and lifestyle choices that support a healthy microbiome, and how gut health enhances metabolic and immune function.

How the Gut Microbiome Influences Immune Response

The gut is often referred to as the body's "second brain," not just because of its intricate neural network but due to its profound impact on immune health. Approximately **70% of the immune system** is housed within the gut, where immune cells interact with the microbiome to regulate inflammation and protect against harmful invaders. When the gut microbiome is in balance, it promotes a strong, regulated immune response. However, when the microbiome is imbalanced—what we call **dysbiosis**—this harmony is disrupted, leading to inflammation and immune dysfunction.

A key component of the gut's defense system is the **intestinal barrier**. This barrier prevents harmful bacteria, toxins, and undigested food particles from entering the bloodstream. A healthy microbiome helps maintain the integrity of this barrier, ensuring that only beneficial nutrients pass through. But when the gut microbiome is disrupted, it weakens the intestinal barrier, allowing toxins and inflammatory compounds to leak into the bloodstream. This condition, known as **leaky gut**, triggers a heightened immune response, causing **systemic inflammation** that can impair metabolic function and increase the risk of developing chronic diseases such as type 2 diabetes and autoimmune disorders.

The gut microbiome also plays a critical role in producing **short-chain fatty acids (SCFAs)**, such as **butyrate**, **acetate**, and **propionate**, which have anti-inflammatory properties. SCFAs are produced when beneficial bacteria ferment fiber in the colon. These compounds help regulate the immune system by promoting the development of **regulatory T cells**, which control inflammation and prevent the immune system from overreacting. By supporting the growth of SCFA-producing bacteria, a balanced microbiome helps reduce chronic inflammation, which is essential for maintaining both metabolic and immune health.

Moreover, the microbiome influences **insulin sensitivity** and overall metabolic function. Certain gut bacteria enhance the body's ability to process glucose, thereby improving insulin sensitivity and reducing the risk of insulin resistance, a precursor to many chronic diseases. When the microbiome is disrupted, however, it can impair blood sugar regulation and contribute to **weight gain**, **metabolic syndrome**, and other related health issues.

Foods and Habits for a Healthy Microbiome

Supporting a healthy gut microbiome is essential for optimizing both metabolic and immune function. The choices you make regarding **diet** and **lifestyle** directly affect the composition and diversity of your gut bacteria. To foster a thriving microbiome, it's important to incorporate habits and foods that promote the growth of beneficial bacteria and minimize factors that contribute to dysbiosis.

One of the most important dietary strategies for supporting a healthy gut is ensuring an adequate intake of **fiber**. As discussed in earlier chapters, fiber acts as a fuel source for the beneficial bacteria in your gut. **Prebiotic fibers**—found in foods like garlic, onions, asparagus, and bananas—specifically help feed **bifidobacteria** and **lactobacilli**, which are associated with improved immune function and reduced inflammation. A varied, fiber-rich diet helps support the production of SCFAs, which further regulate immune responses and promote metabolic health.

In addition to fiber, incorporating **fermented foods** into your diet is a powerful way to introduce beneficial probiotics into the gut. Foods such as **yogurt, kefir, sauerkraut,** and **kimchi** contain live bacteria that help restore balance to the microbiome. These foods can be particularly useful after periods of stress or antibiotic use, which can disrupt the gut's bacterial balance. In some cases, probiotic supplements may also be beneficial, especially when gut health is severely compromised, though it's always ideal to prioritize whole food sources for long-term gut health.

Polyphenols, which are antioxidant compounds found in foods like **green tea, dark chocolate,** and **berries**, also have a positive effect on the gut microbiome. These compounds encourage the growth of beneficial bacteria while inhibiting harmful pathogens. Including polyphenol-rich foods in your diet can help maintain a balanced microbiome and support both immune and metabolic function.

In terms of lifestyle habits, **stress management** is crucial for gut health. As we've previously discussed in Chapters 9 and 3, chronic stress can disrupt the gut's bacterial balance and weaken the integrity of the intestinal barrier. Elevated cortisol levels, caused by long-term stress, are linked to increased inflammation and a decrease in microbial diversity. Incorporating practices such as **meditation, yoga,** and **deep breathing** can help reduce stress and protect the gut from its damaging effects.

While hydration is important for gut function, as we explored in Chapter 2, it's unnecessary to delve into the specifics again here. Instead, let's focus on another key aspect: **sleep**. Poor sleep quality has been shown to negatively affect the microbiome, increasing the risk of dysbiosis. During sleep, the body repairs itself, and this includes maintaining gut health. Consistent, high-quality sleep supports microbial diversity and enhances both metabolic and immune function. As a result, prioritizing a regular sleep routine—aiming for 7-9 hours per night—can have a profound effect on your gut health.

How Gut Health Enhances Metabolic and Immune Function

The gut microbiome plays an essential role in enhancing both **metabolic** and **immune function**, making it a cornerstone of overall health and disease prevention. A well-balanced microbiome not only aids in digestion and nutrient absorption but also helps regulate blood sugar levels, reduce inflammation, and manage fat storage.

One of the ways the microbiome enhances metabolic function is by supporting **insulin sensitivity**. Certain bacteria in the gut produce metabolites that improve how efficiently the body processes glucose. By maintaining a diverse microbiome, you can promote better blood sugar control, which reduces the risk of developing insulin resistance and metabolic disorders like diabetes. On the flip side, an unhealthy microbiome can disrupt this process, leading to poor blood sugar regulation and weight gain.

From an immune perspective, the gut microbiome trains the immune system to differentiate between harmful invaders and the body's own cells. This is particularly important for preventing **autoimmune diseases**, in which the immune system mistakenly attacks healthy tissues. A healthy microbiome promotes **immune tolerance**, helping the body respond appropriately to threats without triggering excessive inflammation or immune dysfunction.

The production of **SCFAs** by beneficial gut bacteria helps control **systemic inflammation**, a major contributor to many chronic diseases. SCFAs promote the development of **regulatory T cells**, which play a critical role in suppressing inflammatory responses. By fostering a microbiome that supports SCFA production, you can help reduce chronic inflammation and improve both immune health and metabolic function.

The microbiome is involved in regulating **hormones**, particularly **cortisol**, the stress hormone. A healthy gut helps moderate the body's stress response, ensuring that cortisol levels don't remain elevated for long periods. This not only reduces stress-related metabolic issues like insulin resistance but also enhances immune resilience.

Chapter 11: Personalized Health and Biohacking

In recent years, medicine has made significant strides toward making health a personalized experience. **Personalized health** focuses on tailoring medical care, lifestyle recommendations, and treatments based on an individual's unique genetic makeup, biometrics, and lifestyle factors. No longer is a one-size-fits-all approach sufficient; the future of health lies in understanding the distinct needs of each individual.

With the rise of **biohacking**, individuals are now empowered to optimize their own health by using data, technology, and self-experimentation. Biohacking goes beyond conventional healthcare and encourages people to actively take control of their metabolic health, energy levels, and overall well-being. From monitoring key health markers to making targeted dietary and lifestyle changes, biohacking offers a proactive way to improve health outcomes.

This chapter will explore the intersection of **personalized medicine** and biohacking, discussing how advancements in genetic testing, biometric tracking, and personalized interventions are revolutionizing the way we approach health. Whether it's through tailoring diets to your specific genetic needs or using wearable technology to optimize daily performance, personalized health and biohacking represent the future of metabolic wellness.

11.1 The Role of Personalized Medicine in Health Optimization

Personalized medicine represents a bold shift in how we approach health, moving from a one-size-fits-all strategy to a tailored approach based on individual biology. The idea behind **personalized medicine** is to use information from your genes, environment, and lifestyle to develop customized health interventions that are more effective and targeted for your unique needs. This approach is particularly powerful for optimizing metabolic health, as genetic differences can significantly affect how we process nutrients, store fat, and respond to exercise.

In this section, we will explore how personalized medicine leverages **genetic testing** to tailor metabolic interventions, how to customize a health plan that matches your biological needs, and the benefits of personalized health assessments.

Using Genetic Testing to Tailor Metabolic Interventions

Genetic testing has become a valuable tool in the realm of personalized health. With advances in technology, we can now decode large sections of our genetic material to gain insights into how our bodies function at a cellular level. This information is critical for understanding individual metabolic responses and crafting personalized interventions that target specific areas where genetic predispositions may cause problems.

For example, genes play a key role in determining **insulin sensitivity, cholesterol metabolism**, and even the way your body handles specific nutrients. Some individuals have genetic variations that make them more prone to **insulin resistance**, while others may metabolize fat less efficiently. These genetic insights allow healthcare providers to tailor **dietary interventions** and **lifestyle recommendations** based on your specific genetic profile.

A gene variant like **FTO**, which is associated with a predisposition to higher body fat, can give healthcare professionals information about how to structure a nutrition and exercise plan that mitigates these effects. Similarly, variations in the **LPL** gene, which affects how the body breaks down fats, may suggest adjustments to dietary fat intake, ensuring that your body efficiently processes the fats you consume.

By using **genetic testing**, we can also identify how your body metabolizes certain vitamins and minerals. For instance, the **MTHFR** gene affects how your body processes folic acid, which can impact energy levels, mood, and overall metabolic function. Armed with this information, health experts can recommend specific supplements or dietary changes to address deficiencies and optimize energy production.

In essence, genetic testing provides the blueprint for your body's metabolic functioning, giving you a clear understanding of which areas may need more support. Instead of following generalized health advice, personalized interventions allow you to focus on what matters most to your specific biology.

Customizing Your Health Plan Based on Unique Biology

Once you've gathered information from genetic testing, the next step is to create a **customized health plan** that aligns with your unique biological needs. Personalization is crucial because it takes into account not only genetic predispositions but also factors such as lifestyle, environment, and personal health goals.

Customizing your plan starts with identifying key areas of metabolic health that need attention. For some, this may involve **improving insulin sensitivity** through a specific exercise routine or adjusting macronutrient ratios. For others, it may be about addressing **chronic inflammation** by reducing foods that trigger inflammatory responses and incorporating more anti-inflammatory nutrients like omega-3 fatty acids.

For individuals who discover they have a genetic predisposition to weight gain or difficulty metabolizing carbohydrates, an effective health plan might include a **low-glycemic index diet**. This would help regulate blood sugar levels, reduce fat storage, and improve energy levels throughout the day. For those with genetic variations that affect **cholesterol metabolism**, focusing on healthy fats like olive oil, nuts, and fatty fish may reduce the risk of cardiovascular issues, improving long-term health outcomes.

Exercise plans can also be customized based on genetic information. If you have a genetic variation that affects how your muscles respond to strength training, your exercise plan might focus more on endurance-based workouts, like cycling or swimming, to optimize cardiovascular health and fat metabolism. If your genes suggest a higher response to **high-intensity interval training (HIIT)**, then a workout plan focusing on short bursts of high-energy exercises may provide faster and more sustainable results.

In addition to diet and exercise, **stress management** and **sleep optimization** are also key elements of a customized health plan. For individuals who are genetically predisposed to higher levels of **cortisol** (the stress hormone), incorporating mindfulness practices, such as meditation or yoga, can help regulate cortisol levels and prevent metabolic disruptions. Meanwhile, understanding how your body responds to **circadian rhythms** can help tailor sleep habits to ensure your body repairs and regenerates efficiently during rest.

Supplements are another area where customization plays a role. Based on genetic testing, you might learn that your body has trouble absorbing certain vitamins or minerals.

For example, those with the **MTHFR gene variant** may require a specific form of **methylated folate** rather than standard folic acid to avoid fatigue and brain fog. Similarly, knowing your body's vitamin D metabolism can help you adjust sun exposure or supplementation to maintain optimal levels for immune function and bone health.

By creating a personalized health plan, you address the unique metabolic and physiological factors that affect your body's performance, enabling you to optimize health outcomes in a way that generalized plans cannot.

Benefits of Personalized Health Assessments

The benefits of adopting a **personalized health assessment** approach are significant, particularly when it comes to metabolic health. By tailoring health interventions based on your genetic makeup and biological needs, you stand to achieve faster and more sustainable results, reducing the risk of chronic diseases and improving quality of life.

One of the main advantages of personalized health assessments is **efficiency**. Instead of guessing which diet, exercise, or supplement regime might work best for you, genetic testing and personalized plans provide clarity. This means that your efforts are more targeted and effective, saving you time and preventing frustration. For instance, if you know that your body responds poorly to high-carbohydrate diets because of genetic predispositions, you can immediately adopt a plan that emphasizes **low-carb**, nutrient-dense meals rather than going through trial and error.

Personalized health assessments also allow for better **preventive care**. Understanding your genetic risks for conditions like **type 2 diabetes**, **heart disease**, or **autoimmune disorders** means that you can take proactive steps to mitigate these risks before they develop into serious health problems. By identifying potential weaknesses in your metabolic health, you can implement strategies to strengthen these areas, whether through diet modifications, supplements, or lifestyle changes.

Another key benefit is the ability to **optimize performance and recovery**. Athletes and fitness enthusiasts, for example, can use genetic insights to fine-tune their training regimens, ensuring they get the best results with minimal risk of injury or burnout. Knowing how your body responds to different forms of exercise, or how it metabolizes nutrients like protein and fat, can help you craft a training and recovery plan that maximizes your gains and keeps you energized throughout the day.

Mental health can also benefit from personalized medicine. Genetic insights into how your body processes **neurotransmitters**—like serotonin and dopamine—can inform strategies for managing stress, anxiety, or depression. By understanding these pathways, you can incorporate specific foods, supplements, and lifestyle changes that support mental well-being alongside physical health.

Finally, personalized health assessments foster a sense of **empowerment**. By gaining a deep understanding of your unique biology, you take control of your health in a more informed and proactive way. Instead of relying on generalized advice, you can implement changes that are specifically designed for your body's needs. This leads to greater confidence in your ability to manage your health and well-being effectively.

11.2 Biohacking for Metabolic Health

Biohacking is an emerging trend that empowers individuals to take control of their own biology by making strategic adjustments to lifestyle, nutrition, and environment. While the term may evoke images of extreme measures or high-tech interventions, at its core, **biohacking** is about using personalized approaches to optimize physical and mental performance, including **metabolic health**. With advances in science and technology, biohacking allows you to track your body's responses to different stimuli and make data-driven decisions to improve energy levels, enhance metabolism, and support overall health.

In this section, we will explore what biohacking is, how it works, and some of the most effective strategies you can use to optimize your metabolic health.

What Biohacking Is and How It Works

At its simplest, **biohacking** involves making intentional, measurable changes to how you eat, sleep, exercise, and manage stress with the goal of enhancing your body's performance. It often incorporates self-experimentation and personalized feedback loops, such as tracking your sleep patterns, blood sugar levels, or energy output, to understand what works best for you. It's about becoming your own health detective, using both traditional wisdom and modern technology to maximize your body's potential.

Many biohackers start by **quantifying their health**—using wearable devices or at-home tests to measure metrics like heart rate variability, blood glucose levels, sleep quality, or even gut health. This data helps you understand how your body responds to certain foods, activities, or environments, allowing you to make adjustments that optimize metabolic efficiency. For example, if you track your blood sugar after meals, you can see how different types of carbohydrates affect your insulin sensitivity and make informed dietary choices based on this information.

Personalization is key to biohacking, and much like personalized medicine, it relies on understanding your unique biological makeup to create a strategy that suits your specific needs. What works for one person might not work for another, and biohacking encourages trial and error to find the best solutions for optimizing health. By experimenting with changes in diet, sleep, exercise, or supplementation, biohackers aim to identify the most effective interventions to boost metabolic health and performance.

Biohacking goes beyond simply making healthy choices—it's about actively testing and refining those choices to achieve the best possible outcomes. Whether you're optimizing energy levels, improving fat metabolism, or boosting cognitive function, biohacking gives you the tools to experiment and adjust your approach based on real-time feedback from your body.

Using Technology to Optimize Energy and Performance

One of the most exciting aspects of biohacking is the use of **technology** to track and improve health metrics. Wearable devices, such as **fitness trackers**, **smartwatches**, and **continuous glucose monitors (CGMs)**, are commonly used in biohacking to monitor various aspects of health and performance. These devices provide valuable data that can be used to optimize metabolic health by adjusting your lifestyle based on what the data reveals.

For example, a **continuous glucose monitor** allows you to track your blood sugar levels throughout the day, giving you real-time insights into how different foods, activities, and stressors impact your blood sugar. By using a CGM, you can see exactly how your body responds to specific meals or snacks, enabling you to make dietary adjustments that improve insulin sensitivity and metabolic function. This approach is particularly valuable for individuals at risk of **insulin resistance** or type 2 diabetes, as it allows for precise, personalized interventions based on real-time data.

Similarly, **sleep trackers** can monitor your sleep cycles, heart rate variability, and even REM stages to provide a detailed picture of your sleep quality. Poor sleep has been shown to disrupt metabolic processes, leading to increased insulin resistance and fat storage. By using sleep-tracking technology, you can make adjustments to your bedtime routine, such as changing your environment or incorporating relaxation techniques, to improve sleep quality and, by extension, your metabolic health.

Heart rate variability (HRV) monitors are another valuable tool in biohacking, particularly for managing stress. HRV measures the variation in time between heartbeats, and it's considered a key indicator of your autonomic nervous system's function. A higher HRV typically indicates better stress resilience and metabolic efficiency. By tracking HRV, you can identify stress triggers and incorporate practices like meditation, yoga, or deep breathing to reduce stress, regulate cortisol levels, and enhance metabolic performance.

In addition to wearable devices, there are also **at-home testing kits** that provide insights into other important aspects of metabolic health, such as **genetic predispositions**, **hormone levels**, or **gut microbiome composition**. These tests allow you to identify areas where your metabolism may be struggling, such as **thyroid function** or **digestive efficiency**, and offer personalized solutions to address those issues.

Biohacking with technology allows for a data-driven approach to improving metabolic health. Instead of relying on generic advice, you can fine-tune your health plan based on metrics unique to your body, ensuring that your interventions are targeted and effective.

Best Biohacks for Improving Metabolic Function

There are many biohacking techniques that can be applied to improve metabolic function, from simple lifestyle changes to more advanced interventions. The key is to start with small, manageable adjustments and build on them as you gather more data about your body's response. Here are some of the most effective biohacks for enhancing metabolic health:

1.   Intermittent Fasting

One of the most popular and well-researched biohacking strategies for metabolic health is **intermittent fasting (IF)**. Intermittent fasting involves cycling between periods of eating and fasting, which has been shown to improve insulin sensitivity, promote fat loss, and enhance mitochondrial function. By giving your body regular breaks from food, you allow it to focus on cellular repair, reduce inflammation, and optimize energy metabolism. Different fasting protocols exist, such as the **16:8 method** (16 hours of fasting followed by an 8-hour eating window), allowing you to choose the approach that works best for your schedule and metabolism.

2.   Cold Exposure

Cold therapy, also known as cold exposure, is another biohack that has gained popularity for its metabolic benefits. Exposing the body to cold temperatures, whether through ice baths, cold showers, or cryotherapy, activates **brown fat**, a type of fat tissue that burns calories to produce heat. Brown fat activation helps boost metabolism and can increase energy expenditure, even when you're at rest. Cold exposure also improves insulin sensitivity and enhances **mitochondrial function**, making it an excellent biohack for those looking to improve metabolic health.

3.   Ketogenic Diet

The **ketogenic diet** is another powerful tool for biohacking metabolic health. By drastically reducing carbohydrate intake and increasing healthy fat consumption, the keto diet encourages the body to enter a state of **ketosis**, where it burns fat for fuel instead of glucose. Ketosis not only promotes fat loss but also improves insulin sensitivity and stabilizes blood sugar levels. Many biohackers use the ketogenic diet to enhance mental clarity, energy levels, and overall metabolic function.

4.   Infrared Sauna Therapy

Infrared saunas have become a popular biohacking tool for improving both metabolic and cardiovascular health. The heat from an infrared sauna penetrates deeper into the body than traditional saunas, promoting detoxification, increasing heart rate, and stimulating **calorie burn**. Regular use of infrared saunas can enhance metabolic function by improving circulation, reducing inflammation, and supporting mitochondrial health.

5.   **Nutrient Timing**

Timing when you eat certain macronutrients—such as carbohydrates, proteins, and fats—can have a significant impact on your metabolism. For example, consuming protein in the morning can help stabilize blood sugar levels throughout the day, while eating carbohydrates post-workout can improve glycogen replenishment and muscle recovery. **Nutrient timing** can be used as a biohacking strategy to enhance energy levels, support fat metabolism, and optimize overall metabolic health.

6.   **Red Light Therapy**

Red light therapy involves exposing the body to low-level wavelengths of red or near-infrared light. This therapy has been shown to improve mitochondrial function, reduce inflammation, and promote faster recovery. Red light therapy can be particularly effective for enhancing fat metabolism, improving skin health, and boosting energy production.

11.3 Tracking Biometrics for Health Improvement

Tracking **biometrics** is a powerful tool for gaining insights into your body's internal processes, especially when it comes to optimizing metabolic health. By gathering data on how your body responds to various stimuli—such as food, exercise, and stress—you can make informed adjustments to your daily routine. These small, data-driven interventions can have a lasting impact on health, helping you achieve improved metabolic function, enhanced energy levels, and better overall well-being. Understanding what metrics to track, how to interpret them, and which tools to use will allow you to create a personalized approach to health optimization.

One of the primary **biometrics** to focus on is **blood glucose**. Monitoring your blood sugar levels provides essential feedback about how well your body processes carbohydrates and regulates insulin. When blood sugar levels spike after a meal, it indicates that the body may not be processing glucose efficiently, which can lead to insulin resistance over time. For those at risk of metabolic disorders, observing these patterns allows you to adjust your diet, focusing on foods that stabilize blood sugar and avoid triggering spikes. Over time, this helps improve **insulin sensitivity** and prevents the onset of chronic conditions like type 2 diabetes.

In addition to blood glucose, understanding **heart rate variability (HRV)** is crucial for tracking stress levels and overall health. HRV measures the variation in time between heartbeats and is a reliable indicator of how well your autonomic nervous system is functioning. Higher HRV typically signals that your body is more resilient to stress, while lower HRV can indicate that stress levels are too high, which can impair metabolic efficiency and immune function. By regularly monitoring HRV, you gain insights into how well your body is coping with stress and can incorporate stress-reducing practices such as meditation or breathing exercises when necessary.

Sleep quality is another biometric closely tied to metabolic health. Poor sleep disrupts hormones, increases insulin resistance, and contributes to fat accumulation, especially around the abdominal area. Tracking sleep patterns—such as the duration of deep sleep and REM cycles—can help you identify areas where your sleep hygiene needs improvement. By optimizing your sleep, you can enhance your body's ability to repair, regulate hormones, and process glucose more effectively, leading to better metabolic outcomes.

Interpreting biometric data requires consistency and attention to trends. It's not just about a single data point; rather, it's about seeing how various metrics evolve over time. For example, if you observe that your blood sugar tends to spike after a specific meal, you can adjust that meal or make changes to how you prepare it. Similarly, if your HRV drops during a particularly stressful week, it might be a signal to incorporate more relaxation techniques into your routine. By tracking these patterns, you become more attuned to your body's signals and can take proactive steps to maintain optimal health.

Several tools and apps are available to make biometric tracking easier and more efficient. Wearable devices, such as **smartwatches** or **fitness trackers**, offer continuous data on heart rate, sleep quality, and activity levels. Some advanced wearables also include HRV monitoring and even track blood oxygen levels, giving a comprehensive view of how well your body is functioning day to day. For those particularly interested in metabolic health, **continuous glucose monitors (CGMs)** are incredibly useful for tracking blood sugar fluctuations throughout the day, allowing real-time feedback on how your diet and lifestyle choices are affecting glucose levels.

Apps that sync with these devices offer helpful interfaces to review and analyze data. You can view trends over days, weeks, or months, and make adjustments accordingly. Some apps even provide personalized recommendations based on the data they collect, helping you refine your approach to nutrition, exercise, and recovery. The power of these tools lies not just in the data they provide, but in how they help you connect the dots between your habits and your health outcomes.

Tracking biometrics also offers a sense of **empowerment**. Rather than relying solely on general advice or periodic medical checkups, you can take daily control of your health by understanding what your body is telling you. Small adjustments based on consistent data can lead to significant improvements over time, reducing the risk of metabolic disorders and enhancing your energy levels and overall performance.

In the end, **tracking biometrics** is about building a clear picture of how your body operates. The more information you have about your body's responses, the better equipped you are to make informed decisions about your health. This leads to a deeper understanding of what helps you thrive, and what might be holding you back, giving you the ability to tailor your lifestyle in ways that optimize metabolic function and support long-term health.

11.4 Nutrigenomics: How Your Diet Affects Your Genes

Nutrigenomics is an exciting field at the intersection of nutrition and genetics, exploring how the foods you eat interact with your genes to influence your overall health. This relatively new area of research highlights the fact that our genes are not static; they can be influenced and expressed differently depending on the environment, especially the nutrients we consume. Understanding your genetic makeup can help you tailor your diet to optimize **metabolic health**, improve energy levels, and reduce the risk of developing chronic conditions.

In this section, we'll dive into how **nutrigenomics** works, the science behind how diet affects gene expression, and how to customize your diet based on genetic insights for optimal health outcomes.

The Science Behind Nutrigenomics

At the heart of **nutrigenomics** is the concept of **gene expression**, which refers to how active or inactive certain genes are in determining your body's functions. Although you inherit your genetic code from your parents, not all genes are active all the time. Specific environmental factors, including the nutrients you consume, can "switch on" or "switch off" certain genes, impacting how your body functions at a cellular level. This means that while you may have a genetic predisposition to certain health conditions, your diet has the potential to influence whether those genes are expressed.

One of the best-known examples of nutrigenomics in action is how dietary fat intake affects individuals with variations in the **APOE gene**, which is linked to cholesterol metabolism. Those with certain variations of the APOE gene are more sensitive to saturated fats, and consuming high amounts can increase their risk of cardiovascular disease. In this case, understanding your genetic makeup can lead to more personalized dietary recommendations, helping individuals reduce their risk of heart disease by limiting saturated fat intake and prioritizing healthier fats, such as those found in olive oil and avocados.

Similarly, the way your body processes certain vitamins, minerals, and other nutrients can also be influenced by your genes. For instance, individuals with specific variants of the **MTHFR gene** may have a reduced ability to convert folic acid into its active form, methylfolate, which plays a crucial role in DNA synthesis, cell repair, and detoxification processes. For these individuals, consuming foods rich in natural folate or taking supplements with methylated folate can make a significant difference in their overall metabolic health and energy levels.

Another example lies in how some people are genetically predisposed to **insulin resistance** or have a higher risk of developing type 2 diabetes. By understanding their genetic profile, they can proactively adjust their diet to avoid excessive carbohydrates and sugars, which may exacerbate their condition. Instead, they can focus on a diet rich in whole foods, lean proteins, healthy fats, and fiber to maintain stable blood sugar levels and support metabolic function.

Customizing Your Diet Based on Genetic Information

The ultimate goal of nutrigenomics is to help individuals create a **personalized diet** that optimizes health by taking into account their unique genetic profile. After undergoing genetic testing, which is increasingly available through at-home kits or professional healthcare providers, you can use the insights gained to adjust your nutritional approach in ways that target your metabolic health more effectively.

For example, if your genetic results indicate that you are prone to inflammation, you can modify your diet to include more **anti-inflammatory foods**, such as fatty fish, leafy greens, and berries, while avoiding pro-inflammatory foods like processed meats and refined sugars. This approach helps minimize the activation of genes that promote inflammation, thereby protecting you from chronic conditions such as heart disease, diabetes, and autoimmune disorders.

Another scenario might involve individuals who metabolize caffeine differently due to variations in the **CYP1A2 gene**, which affects how quickly caffeine is processed in the liver. Those with a "slow" metabolism of caffeine may experience increased anxiety, higher blood pressure, or disrupted sleep when consuming even moderate amounts of caffeine. Armed with this knowledge, they can adjust their coffee or tea consumption to avoid these side effects and maintain optimal energy and focus.

The power of nutrigenomics lies in its ability to offer **precision nutrition**—a highly targeted approach to diet that acknowledges genetic individuality. Instead of following broad dietary guidelines, you can create a nutrition plan that aligns with your biological needs. This means you're more likely to experience positive health outcomes, as your diet will work with your body's natural genetic tendencies rather than against them.

Furthermore, nutrigenomics can guide supplementation strategies. Genetic testing can reveal if you're predisposed to deficiencies in certain vitamins or minerals, allowing you to take specific supplements tailored to your needs. For example, those with the **FUT2 gene variant** may have a reduced ability to absorb vitamin B12, even if they're consuming adequate amounts in their diet. In such cases, a targeted supplement plan can help address this deficiency and support metabolic health and energy levels.

Nutrient timing is another factor influenced by genetics. Some individuals may be genetically predisposed to perform better with smaller, more frequent meals that maintain stable blood sugar levels, while others may thrive on intermittent fasting, where the timing of food intake is restricted to certain windows during the day. Genetic testing can reveal these tendencies, allowing you to choose the eating pattern that best suits your metabolism.

How Your Genetic Makeup Influences Dietary Needs

It's important to understand that while genes play a significant role in determining how you respond to various nutrients, they are not the sole factor. Your **lifestyle**, including your physical activity level, stress management, and sleep quality, also contributes to how well your body processes food and nutrients. However, knowing your genetic predispositions gives you a critical advantage in making smarter dietary decisions.

For instance, individuals who carry a variation of the **FTO gene**—often referred to as the "fat mass and obesity-associated gene"—may be more likely to gain weight when consuming a diet high in carbohydrates and fats. This knowledge allows for preemptive adjustments to their diet, such as prioritizing a higher-protein, lower-carbohydrate diet that supports lean muscle mass and fat loss. By understanding how the FTO gene interacts with dietary choices, individuals can take proactive steps to avoid excessive weight gain and metabolic disorders.

Another gene that plays a role in dietary needs is **SLC2A9**, which affects uric acid metabolism and can predispose individuals to conditions like **gout** when purine-rich foods are consumed in excess. Knowing about this genetic risk can prompt you to limit foods like red meat and certain seafood that are high in purines, preventing flare-ups and promoting overall metabolic health.

Nutrigenomics also emphasizes the importance of **food quality**. For example, some people may have genes that make them more sensitive to environmental toxins or pesticide residues found in conventionally grown produce. In such cases, choosing **organic produce** and minimizing exposure to toxins can help reduce the risk of triggering genetic pathways associated with inflammation and metabolic dysfunction.

11.5 Building a Personalized Health Routine

Crafting a **personalized health routine** is essential to optimize your overall well-being by incorporating the insights gained from both personalized medicine and biohacking strategies. Unlike generic health plans, a personalized routine is tailored to your unique genetic makeup, lifestyle, and health goals. It takes into account not only your metabolic tendencies but also how your body responds to various factors like nutrition, physical activity, sleep, and stress management.

In this section, we'll explore how to build an effective and sustainable health routine based on personalized insights, how to incorporate biohacking practices into your daily life, and why adaptability is crucial as your needs evolve over time.

Steps to Create a Health Plan Tailored to You

The foundation of a personalized health routine begins with understanding your **unique biology**. Whether through genetic testing, biometric monitoring, or simply paying closer attention to how your body reacts to different lifestyle factors, the first step is gathering data that informs your health decisions. Armed with this information, you can design a routine that supports your metabolic health and fits seamlessly into your daily life.

Start by prioritizing key areas that directly impact your health, such as **nutrition, exercise, sleep**, and **stress management**. For each of these components, tailor your routine based on the data you've collected. If your genetic profile indicates a predisposition to **insulin resistance**, for example, focusing on low-glycemic foods and maintaining steady blood sugar levels throughout the day is vital. This might mean planning meals rich in fiber, protein, and healthy fats, avoiding refined sugars, and incorporating intermittent fasting if your body responds well to it.

For **physical activity**, consider how your body's specific needs dictate the type of exercise that will provide the most benefit. If your biometrics suggest a lower capacity for high-intensity exercises but a good response to endurance training, building a routine around longer, moderate activities like walking, swimming, or cycling will help improve metabolic efficiency without causing burnout. Conversely, those whose metrics favor strength training or **high-intensity interval training (HIIT)** can incorporate those exercises into their plan to maximize results.

Once you have a structure in place, it's essential to **listen to your body's feedback**. The key to personalizing a health routine is continuous adaptation. Your body's needs can shift over time due to factors like aging, hormonal changes, or evolving stress levels, and your routine should reflect these changes. By periodically assessing how your body responds to different elements of your routine, such as dietary changes or new fitness plans, you can refine and adjust as necessary.

Integrating Biohacking Practices Into Daily Life

Biohacking offers numerous ways to fine-tune your routine to meet your goals more effectively. While it might seem like a complicated, tech-driven approach, biohacking can be simplified into practical actions you can easily integrate into your life.

One of the simplest biohacking techniques to start with is **tracking biometrics**. Whether through wearable devices or simple apps that track your diet and sleep, gathering data on your daily habits provides a deeper understanding of what's working and where improvements can be made. For example, using a **sleep tracker** to monitor the quality of your rest can help you determine whether adjustments to your sleep environment are necessary. If your sleep metrics consistently show poor recovery or interrupted cycles, making changes to your bedroom—like minimizing light exposure or reducing noise—can lead to better sleep quality, which in turn improves metabolic function.

Another powerful biohacking tool is **continuous glucose monitoring (CGM)**, which allows you to observe how specific foods and activities affect your blood sugar levels in real time. This feedback is invaluable for fine-tuning your diet. You may discover that certain meals cause blood sugar spikes, prompting you to modify ingredients or portion sizes to keep your glucose levels stable. Over time, you can optimize your dietary choices to support better energy levels and prevent insulin resistance, ultimately enhancing your metabolic health.

Incorporating **intermittent fasting** can also be a beneficial biohacking practice. By restricting your eating window and allowing your body to enter a fasting state, you promote cellular repair and improve insulin sensitivity. If your health data suggests a predisposition to weight gain or insulin resistance, experimenting with intermittent fasting may provide a simple but effective way to manage these issues.

Another effective biohack is **cold exposure** therapy, which can be as simple as ending your showers with cold water or taking brief ice baths. Cold exposure activates **brown fat**, which burns calories to generate heat and has been shown to improve metabolism and insulin sensitivity. Additionally, cold therapy can help reduce inflammation and enhance recovery after physical activity, making it a useful tool for those aiming to improve both metabolic and physical performance.

By integrating these biohacking techniques into your routine, you can experiment with small adjustments and gather data to see which interventions have the most significant impact on your health. Biohacking is about using measurable results to guide your health decisions, making it a perfect complement to a personalized health plan.

Adapting Your Routine as Your Needs Evolve

Building a personalized health routine is not a one-time process. Over time, as your body changes and your health goals shift, your routine should evolve to meet those needs. Flexibility is crucial when it comes to personalizing your health approach.

Regularly reassessing your biometric data allows you to make informed adjustments. For example, if you notice that your **heart rate variability (HRV)** is declining, indicating higher stress levels, it might be time to adjust your stress management techniques, incorporating more relaxation or mindfulness practices. Similarly, if your sleep quality starts to degrade, revisiting your sleep hygiene and making changes to improve your rest will be essential for maintaining your metabolic health.

Age also plays a critical role in how your body responds to diet and exercise. As you get older, your metabolism may slow, and recovery times from physical activity might lengthen. In these cases, you may need to adjust your routine to include more **restorative practices**, such as yoga or stretching, alongside your regular workouts. Additionally, focusing on nutrition that supports **joint health**, **bone density**, and **muscle mass** becomes more important as you age.

Hormonal shifts, especially during major life changes such as pregnancy, menopause, or aging, may also require adjustments to your routine. For women going through menopause, prioritizing foods rich in **phytoestrogens** (such as flaxseeds and soy products) may help balance hormonal fluctuations, while incorporating **resistance training** can preserve muscle mass and improve metabolic function.

Moreover, your environment can influence how your health routine should evolve. If you move to a new location with a different climate or altitude, your body may respond differently to the same activities or foods. Paying attention to these environmental shifts and adapting accordingly ensures that your routine remains effective in supporting metabolic health and overall well-being.

The ability to remain flexible and adapt your routine over time is key to maintaining long-term success. Your personalized health plan should be a living strategy, constantly evolving based on new information, feedback from your body, and changes in your life circumstances.

Chapter 12: Future Trends in Health and Metabolism

As we conclude this journey, it's time to turn our attention to the future. The world of health and metabolism is evolving rapidly, and with it, the opportunities for **optimizing metabolic health** are becoming more sophisticated and personalized. While you've learned a great deal about how to manage and improve your metabolism throughout this book, the next frontier promises even more powerful tools and insights. In this final chapter, we'll explore the emerging trends, scientific breakthroughs, and the role of technology in the future of metabolic research and health optimization.

12.1 The Future of Metabolic Research

Metabolism is the cornerstone of health, and the future of metabolic research is poised to bring revolutionary changes in how we understand and treat metabolic function. As science continues to delve into the complexities of cellular energy production, inflammation, and genetic expression, we're on the verge of groundbreaking discoveries that will change the way we approach health and disease prevention.

Emerging Science in Metabolic Health

One of the most exciting areas of future research involves **metabolic flexibility**, which refers to the body's ability to seamlessly switch between using carbohydrates and fats as fuel. Metabolic flexibility is essential for maintaining energy levels, weight management, and preventing insulin resistance. However, many people today, due to poor diet and sedentary lifestyles, suffer from poor metabolic flexibility, making them more prone to energy crashes, weight gain, and metabolic disorders. Emerging research aims to explore how specific dietary interventions, exercise routines, and possibly pharmaceuticals can enhance metabolic flexibility, making it easier to burn fat for energy while stabilizing blood sugar levels.

Another focus area is the role of **mitochondria**—the energy-producing powerhouses of our cells—in metabolic health. Research is revealing new ways to optimize mitochondrial function to improve energy production, reduce oxidative stress, and prevent mitochondrial dysfunction, which is linked to metabolic disorders, aging, and even neurodegenerative diseases. **Mitochondrial biogenesis**, the process of creating new mitochondria, is becoming a target for therapies aimed at boosting metabolic health and delaying age-related decline. Scientists are looking into both nutritional and pharmaceutical interventions to support mitochondrial health and improve overall metabolic function.

Epigenetics is another promising field. It explores how environmental factors—like diet, exercise, and even stress—affect the way our genes are expressed. While your genetic code doesn't change, epigenetics shows us that gene expression can be modified to improve or impair metabolic function. As this area of research grows, personalized interventions based on your epigenetic profile may become more accessible, allowing for diet and lifestyle recommendations that enhance **insulin sensitivity**, reduce inflammation, and optimize energy metabolism.

Lastly, research into the **gut microbiome** and its link to metabolism continues to expand. Scientists are discovering that certain strains of gut bacteria can either improve or impair metabolic health. Future breakthroughs could lead to targeted probiotics or even **microbiome transplants** to correct imbalances, allowing individuals to optimize their microbiota for better glucose regulation, fat metabolism, and reduced inflammation.

Breakthroughs in Treating Metabolic Disorders

One of the most significant areas of focus in metabolic research is the treatment of **metabolic disorders** such as **type 2 diabetes, obesity**, and **metabolic syndrome**. While lifestyle changes remain the first line of defense against these conditions, future treatments will likely include more personalized and precise interventions. Scientists are working on **gene therapies** that could correct genetic predispositions to insulin resistance or obesity, fundamentally altering how we treat these disorders.

There is also ongoing research into the use of **pharmacological agents** that target specific metabolic pathways. For example, certain drugs may soon be available to help increase **insulin sensitivity** without the side effects of current medications. These treatments will focus on improving the body's ability to manage blood sugar levels more efficiently, potentially reversing early-stage metabolic disorders before they lead to more severe conditions.

In addition, advances in **weight loss medications** are on the horizon. While traditional approaches to weight management often focus on diet and exercise alone, new medications are being developed to regulate appetite, improve fat metabolism, and increase energy expenditure. These drugs are expected to provide safer, more effective options for those struggling with obesity-related metabolic issues.

Another promising breakthrough is in the field of **regenerative medicine**, where researchers are exploring the potential of **stem cell therapy** to repair damaged tissues and organs affected by metabolic dysfunction. For instance, in type 1 and type 2 diabetes, stem cell treatments may one day help regenerate insulin-producing cells in the pancreas, offering a potential cure rather than just managing symptoms.

Technology's Role in Health Optimization

The future of metabolic health will be heavily influenced by **technology**, with tools that allow for real-time monitoring, precision interventions, and more personalized care becoming more widespread. As wearables, AI, and data analytics continue to improve, individuals will have more control than ever over their metabolic health.

Wearable technology, such as continuous glucose monitors (CGMs) and smartwatches, will continue to evolve, offering even more precise insights into how your body responds to food, activity, and stress. These devices already track real-time data on blood sugar levels, sleep patterns, and heart rate variability, but future iterations will likely provide even deeper insights into **hormone levels**, **mitochondrial function**, and other key biomarkers of metabolic health. This data will help individuals fine-tune their diet and exercise plans to optimize metabolism in real time.

Artificial intelligence (AI) and **machine learning** will play a significant role in this evolution as well. AI-driven apps and platforms will be able to analyze your personal health data—ranging from genetic tests to biometric monitoring—and provide tailored recommendations for nutrition, exercise, and stress management. These recommendations will not be based on general guidelines but on your specific biological needs, making health optimization more accessible and effective for everyone.

AI will also be integral in **personalized medicine** as it analyzes large datasets from clinical trials, patient histories, and genetic profiles to predict which treatments will work best for specific individuals. In the future, you may receive personalized medication plans or nutritional advice generated by AI based on your unique genetic makeup, medical history, and lifestyle habits. This approach will reduce the trial-and-error period currently required for finding effective treatments and allow for faster, more targeted health interventions.

Telemedicine and **remote health monitoring** will become even more integral to optimizing metabolic health. Instead of relying on annual doctor visits or lab tests, individuals will be able to share their real-time health data with their healthcare providers through secure platforms. This allows for ongoing adjustments to their health plans based on how they're responding to treatment or lifestyle changes. Remote monitoring, paired with personalized AI-driven health recommendations, means that metabolic health can be managed more proactively than ever before, potentially preventing chronic conditions from developing or worsening.

12.2 The Role of Artificial Intelligence in Healthcare

As technology advances, **artificial intelligence (AI)** is increasingly playing a transformative role in healthcare, particularly in the realm of **metabolic health**. AI's ability to analyze vast amounts of data quickly and accurately has opened up new possibilities for personalized medicine, health monitoring, and predictive care. With AI, healthcare is becoming more precise, targeted, and individualized, offering better outcomes for patients by tailoring interventions to their unique biological needs.

In this section, we'll explore how AI is revolutionizing metabolic health through **diagnosis and treatment, personalized health recommendations**, and its future impact on **metabolic interventions**.

How AI Is Transforming Diagnosis and Treatment

Traditionally, diagnosing metabolic disorders like diabetes, obesity, or metabolic syndrome involves a range of tests, assessments, and clinical judgments that rely on established medical guidelines. While effective, these methods can be slow and imprecise, particularly when dealing with complex cases or subtle early-stage conditions. AI is changing this by offering faster, more accurate diagnostic capabilities.

One of AI's greatest strengths lies in its ability to **analyze large datasets** of patient information, including genetic profiles, medical histories, lifestyle data, and biomarkers. By processing this data, AI algorithms can identify patterns and correlations that would be impossible for a human clinician to detect. For example, AI can analyze continuous glucose monitoring (CGM) data to identify patterns of insulin resistance or blood sugar fluctuations long before a patient might be diagnosed with type 2 diabetes. By catching these signs early, AI can help healthcare providers intervene before a condition progresses into something more serious.

In the realm of treatment, AI is also changing the game. With access to vast amounts of clinical trial data, patient outcomes, and research, AI can help **predict which treatments** or lifestyle interventions will be most effective for individual patients. This capability allows for more targeted, personalized care. For instance, rather than starting a patient on a standard treatment for metabolic syndrome, AI can analyze the patient's genetic and lifestyle data to recommend a medication or dietary change specifically tailored to their unique needs.

AI is also beginning to make its way into **surgical interventions** for metabolic conditions like obesity. Advanced robotic surgery systems powered by AI are becoming more precise, offering less invasive options with shorter recovery times. This technology is helping improve outcomes for procedures like gastric bypass surgery, which is often used as a last-resort treatment for severe metabolic disorders.

Personalized Health Recommendations Powered by AI

Perhaps the most exciting application of AI in metabolic health is its ability to generate **personalized health recommendations**. Traditional health advice tends to follow generalized guidelines, which don't always work for everyone. What AI offers is a way to tailor these recommendations to the specific needs of the individual, taking into account factors like **genetic predispositions**, **biometric data**, **dietary habits**, and **lifestyle**.

AI-powered health apps and platforms are already making strides in this direction. These tools analyze your health data in real time, offering customized recommendations for diet, exercise, and lifestyle adjustments that align with your unique metabolic profile. For example, an AI-driven app could analyze your continuous glucose monitoring data and suggest adjustments to your daily meals based on how your body processes carbohydrates. It might recommend a lower-carb breakfast after detecting a spike in your blood sugar from a high-carb meal the previous day, or suggest a post-workout snack that aligns with your metabolism's needs for better recovery.

AI can also assess patterns over time, detecting subtle changes in your health that might not be apparent through traditional monitoring. For instance, if an AI system detects that your **heart rate variability (HRV)** is consistently low—an indication of elevated stress—it might recommend stress-relief techniques such as meditation or deep breathing exercises, and track how these interventions affect your overall metabolic health. Similarly, if sleep metrics show signs of poor recovery, AI can suggest modifications to your **sleep hygiene**, recommending adjustments to bedtime routines or environmental factors like light exposure and room temperature.

With AI constantly analyzing your health metrics, it can deliver **real-time feedback** to help you optimize your health decisions. Over time, these personalized recommendations can improve metabolic efficiency, helping to prevent the development of metabolic disorders and enhancing your quality of life.

The Future of AI-Driven Metabolic Interventions

As AI continues to evolve, its potential to revolutionize metabolic health goes far beyond current applications. One of the most exciting areas of development is the integration of **AI with precision medicine**. AI has the ability to integrate data from genetic testing, epigenetics, and real-time biometrics to create fully customized health interventions. This level of precision will not only improve metabolic health but could also help **prevent diseases** long before they manifest.

For example, AI could predict an individual's risk of developing type 2 diabetes or heart disease based on a combination of genetic markers and real-time data, such as **blood sugar levels**, **dietary habits**, and **activity levels**. With this information, AI could recommend a highly targeted intervention—whether it's a specific type of exercise, a personalized diet plan, or a tailored medication regimen—that is designed to prevent the condition from ever taking root. This predictive approach could transform healthcare from a reactive model to a proactive one, helping individuals maintain their metabolic health well into old age.

AI's potential in pharmacogenomics—how your genetic makeup affects your response to medications—will also play a significant role in metabolic health. By analyzing a patient's genetic profile, AI can predict which medications will work best for them and at what dosage, reducing the trial-and-error period that often accompanies drug prescriptions. This is particularly useful for treating metabolic disorders, where finding the right medication or combination of treatments can take time. AI-driven insights will help doctors prescribe **precision medications** that are more effective and have fewer side effects.

Another promising area is **AI-powered wearables**. As wearable devices become more sophisticated, they will integrate AI to provide real-time insights that can significantly enhance metabolic function. These devices could monitor not only heart rate, glucose levels, and sleep patterns but also track **hormonal fluctuations, inflammatory markers**, and **gut microbiome activity**. AI would then process all of this information and recommend interventions that optimize metabolic health down to the cellular level.

In the future, **AI-guided therapies** may also extend to optimizing mitochondrial function, reducing oxidative stress, and even delaying the effects of aging. AI could analyze mitochondrial health and recommend targeted therapies such as **red light therapy**, specific nutrients, or even **mitochondrial biogenesis** boosters to enhance cellular energy production and metabolic efficiency.

The integration of AI in metabolic health will also change how we approach chronic disease management. By continuously monitoring patients and providing **adaptive health plans**, AI will make managing conditions like diabetes or cardiovascular disease much more seamless. Patients will receive real-time insights into their condition, allowing them to adjust medications, diets, or activity levels as needed to maintain balance.

12.3 Advances in Genetic Engineering for Health

As our understanding of genetics deepens, **genetic engineering** is emerging as one of the most exciting frontiers in healthcare. The ability to manipulate genes and edit DNA holds incredible promise for improving **metabolic health** and addressing a wide range of diseases, from obesity and diabetes to more complex metabolic disorders. With groundbreaking technologies like **CRISPR** and **gene therapy**, genetic engineering is poised to revolutionize not only how we treat diseases but also how we prevent them. In this section, we'll explore the latest advancements in genetic engineering and how they may shape the future of metabolic health.

CRISPR and Its Role in Future Health Innovations

One of the most significant developments in genetic engineering is **CRISPR-Cas9** technology, a tool that allows scientists to precisely edit genes. CRISPR (Clustered Regularly Interspaced Short Palindromic Repeats) is essentially a molecular "scissor" that can target and modify specific genes within DNA, offering the potential to correct genetic mutations that lead to diseases. This technology is already being used in experimental treatments for genetic disorders like cystic fibrosis and sickle cell anemia, but its application to metabolic health is just beginning.

In the context of metabolic disorders, CRISPR could be used to **alter genes** that predispose individuals to conditions like **type 2 diabetes**, **obesity**, or **insulin resistance**. For example, researchers are exploring how to modify the **FTO gene**, which has been linked to higher body fat and obesity. By editing this gene, scientists could potentially reduce an individual's risk of developing obesity and its related metabolic complications. Similarly, **genes involved in cholesterol metabolism**, like **PCSK9**, could be edited to lower cholesterol levels and reduce the risk of heart disease.

Another promising area for CRISPR is in the treatment of **monogenic metabolic disorders**, which are diseases caused by a single genetic mutation. Conditions like **familial hypercholesterolemia**, which leads to extremely high cholesterol levels, or **Prader-Willi syndrome**, which affects appetite and metabolism, could potentially be cured by correcting the underlying genetic mutation. By targeting the specific gene responsible for the disorder, CRISPR offers a more permanent and precise solution than current treatments, which often only manage symptoms.

While CRISPR's potential is immense, it is not without challenges. Ethical considerations, such as the possibility of unintended genetic changes or "off-target" effects, need to be carefully addressed. However, as the technology advances and becomes more refined, CRISPR is expected to play a central role in **genetic therapies** for metabolic and other chronic health conditions.

How Genetic Engineering Could Address Metabolic Diseases

Beyond CRISPR, other forms of **gene therapy** are being developed to treat and prevent metabolic diseases. Gene therapy involves introducing, removing, or altering genetic material in a person's cells to treat or prevent disease. While still in its early stages, gene therapy has the potential to **modify how genes are expressed**, offering a new way to address the root causes of metabolic conditions rather than just managing their symptoms.

For example, **gene therapy for diabetes** could involve altering genes in **pancreatic beta cells**, enabling them to produce insulin more effectively. This would be especially impactful for people with **type 1 diabetes**, where the immune system destroys insulin-producing cells. Scientists are also exploring how to use gene therapy to improve insulin sensitivity, which could reduce the need for medication and lifestyle interventions in people with **type 2 diabetes**.

In obesity treatment, genetic engineering could target genes that regulate **appetite**, **energy expenditure**, or **fat storage**. By altering the expression of these genes, it might be possible to create a long-term solution for managing weight. For instance, researchers are investigating how to **increase brown fat activity** (brown fat burns calories to generate heat) or **reduce the efficiency of white fat storage** (white fat stores excess energy) through genetic modification.

One of the most promising areas of research is in the treatment of **genetic metabolic disorders** like **phenylketonuria (PKU)** and **Gaucher disease**. These disorders occur when genetic mutations prevent the body from processing certain nutrients properly, leading to toxic buildups and serious health complications. Gene therapy could correct these mutations, allowing patients to live normal, healthy lives without the need for restrictive diets or enzyme replacement therapies.

Gene therapies for metabolic diseases could also extend beyond just correcting mutations. Scientists are exploring ways to **enhance certain genetic functions** to improve metabolic efficiency, reduce inflammation, and prevent the onset of chronic diseases. For example, by upregulating genes that improve **mitochondrial function**, gene therapy could help increase energy production at the cellular level, potentially delaying the aging process and preventing age-related metabolic decline.

Ethical Considerations Around Genetic Health Interventions

As promising as genetic engineering is, it brings with it significant **ethical concerns**. The ability to edit genes, especially in ways that could be inherited by future generations, raises questions about the long-term impacts on humanity. Some fear that genetic editing could lead to "designer babies," where genetic modifications are used for cosmetic or non-essential purposes rather than medical ones.

In the context of metabolic health, the ethical questions are a bit more focused on how to ensure that these therapies are safe and accessible. Editing genes related to **metabolism**, for example, could have far-reaching effects on a person's overall physiology. While improving insulin sensitivity or reducing fat storage may seem straightforward, we must also consider the **long-term consequences** of such modifications. Could these changes affect other aspects of health? Could they unintentionally impact lifespan or fertility? As genetic engineering becomes more widespread, researchers will need to ensure that the risks are thoroughly understood and that patients are fully informed.

Another major ethical consideration is **accessibility**. Genetic engineering technologies are likely to be expensive, at least initially. This raises concerns about **health equity**—will only the wealthy be able to afford treatments that could prevent or cure metabolic diseases? Ensuring that these groundbreaking therapies are available to everyone, regardless of socioeconomic status, will be a critical issue as they become more common.

There is also the issue of **genetic privacy**. As more individuals undergo genetic testing and therapy, the potential for misuse of genetic information grows. Privacy laws will need to evolve to protect individuals from discrimination based on their genetic profile, particularly as it relates to metabolic health and conditions like diabetes, obesity, and cardiovascular disease.

12.4 Longevity and Metabolic Function

As research into health and wellness progresses, a growing body of evidence suggests that **metabolic health** is deeply tied to **longevity**. In the pursuit of a longer, healthier life, understanding and optimizing metabolic processes becomes crucial. The future of metabolic health is not just about preventing diseases like diabetes or heart disease but also about **extending lifespan** and improving **healthspan**—the number of years we live in good health.

In this section, we'll explore the connection between metabolic function and longevity, how advances in longevity research are impacting metabolic health, and practical steps you can take to support **long-term metabolic vitality**.

The Connection Between Optimized Metabolism and Extended Lifespan

One of the most significant factors influencing lifespan is the body's ability to efficiently convert food into energy while minimizing the negative effects of that process, such as **oxidative stress** and **inflammation**. **Mitochondria**, the energy producers within our cells, play a central role in this process. As we age, mitochondrial function declines, leading to reduced energy production, increased oxidative damage, and metabolic inefficiency. This decline in mitochondrial health is linked to many age-related diseases, including heart disease, neurodegenerative conditions, and metabolic disorders like type 2 diabetes.

Optimizing mitochondrial function is a key strategy for promoting longevity. Advances in research are showing that **enhancing mitochondrial efficiency**—either through lifestyle interventions, supplements, or emerging therapies—can slow down the aging process and improve metabolic health. For example, practices like **intermittent fasting** and **caloric restriction** have been shown to promote mitochondrial biogenesis (the creation of new mitochondria), improve insulin sensitivity, and reduce oxidative stress. These benefits contribute to both longer lifespan and better metabolic function over time.

Another critical aspect of metabolism and longevity is **insulin sensitivity**. Insulin resistance, which impairs the body's ability to manage blood sugar, is a major contributor to the development of chronic diseases and a shortened lifespan. By maintaining stable blood sugar levels and improving insulin sensitivity, you reduce the risk of diseases such as

type 2 diabetes, heart disease, and obesity, which can all negatively impact longevity. Strategies to improve insulin sensitivity include regular physical activity, maintaining a balanced diet, and possibly the use of specific supplements that support glucose metabolism.

In addition to insulin sensitivity and mitochondrial health, the role of **inflammation** cannot be ignored. Chronic low-grade inflammation, often referred to as **inflammaging**, accelerates the aging process and impairs metabolic function. Reducing systemic inflammation through **anti-inflammatory diets**, regular physical activity, and stress management techniques can promote both better metabolic health and a longer lifespan.

How Advances in Longevity Research Impact Metabolic Health

The field of **longevity research** is rapidly evolving, and many of the breakthroughs in this area have direct implications for metabolic health. **Caloric restriction** and **fasting-mimicking diets** are two areas that have garnered a lot of attention due to their effects on metabolic processes and lifespan extension. Both approaches have been shown to improve metabolic efficiency, reduce oxidative stress, and trigger cellular repair mechanisms like **autophagy**, where cells remove damaged components, enhancing overall metabolic health.

Researchers are also exploring **senolytics**, a class of compounds designed to target and eliminate **senescent cells**—cells that have stopped dividing but remain in the body, contributing to inflammation and tissue damage. By clearing out these senescent cells, senolytics have the potential to reduce age-related inflammation and improve metabolic function, thus promoting longevity. Early studies in animals have shown promise, and human trials are underway to explore the effects of senolytic therapies on aging and metabolic health.

Another promising area of longevity research involves **NAD+ (nicotinamide adenine dinucleotide)**, a molecule critical for cellular energy production and mitochondrial function. As we age, NAD+ levels decline, leading to decreased mitochondrial efficiency and impaired metabolic health. Supplementing with NAD+ precursors, such as **nicotinamide riboside (NR)** or **nicotinamide mononucleotide (NMN)**, has been shown to boost NAD+ levels, enhance mitochondrial function, and improve metabolic processes. These compounds are currently being studied for their potential to extend lifespan and promote healthy aging by optimizing metabolism at the cellular level.

Stem cell research is another area impacting metabolic health and longevity. As we age, the body's ability to regenerate tissue and repair damage declines, leading to metabolic inefficiencies and a higher risk of disease. Advances in stem cell therapies aim to rejuvenate the body's regenerative capacity, potentially improving metabolic health and extending both lifespan and healthspan.

Genetic engineering and **CRISPR** technologies offer exciting possibilities for correcting metabolic dysfunctions at the genetic level. By targeting genes related to metabolism, researchers may one day be able to eliminate genetic predispositions to insulin resistance, obesity, or other metabolic conditions that shorten lifespan. While this technology is still in its early stages, it holds immense promise for the future of personalized medicine and longevity.

Practical Steps to Improve Longevity Through Metabolic Balance

While advances in longevity research are exciting, there are practical steps you can take today to optimize your metabolic health and support a longer, healthier life. Many of the strategies discussed throughout this book—such as maintaining a balanced diet, incorporating regular exercise, managing stress, and prioritizing sleep—are foundational for both metabolic health and longevity.

One of the most effective ways to support longevity is through **intermittent fasting** or **time-restricted eating**, which encourages metabolic flexibility, enhances mitochondrial function, and promotes autophagy. By giving your body extended periods without food, you allow it to focus on repair processes rather than constantly digesting food, which helps preserve metabolic health over the long term.

Another important factor is **muscle mass**. As we age, muscle mass naturally declines, leading to a slower metabolism and an increased risk of metabolic diseases. Strength training and resistance exercises are crucial for maintaining muscle mass, improving insulin sensitivity, and supporting metabolic health. In addition, maintaining lean muscle helps improve fat metabolism and contributes to a more active, healthy lifestyle well into old age.

Nutritional strategies are also key. Prioritizing **anti-inflammatory foods** such as leafy greens, fatty fish, and berries helps reduce systemic inflammation, a major contributor to both metabolic dysfunction and aging. Incorporating **healthy fats**, like those found in olive oil, nuts, and avocados, supports heart health and metabolic function. Limiting refined sugars and processed carbohydrates helps prevent insulin resistance, a significant factor in accelerated aging and metabolic disorders.

Stress management is critical for both metabolic health and longevity. Chronic stress contributes to elevated cortisol levels, which can lead to insulin resistance, weight gain, and increased inflammation—all of which impair metabolic health. Practices like **mindfulness**, **meditation**, and **deep breathing** can help reduce stress, lower cortisol levels, and support a balanced metabolic state that promotes longevity.

The connection between **longevity** and **metabolic function** is becoming clearer with ongoing research. As we continue to uncover new ways to optimize metabolism through both lifestyle interventions and emerging technologies, the potential to extend lifespan while improving healthspan is becoming more achievable. By focusing on mitochondrial health, reducing inflammation, improving insulin sensitivity, and integrating the latest findings from longevity research, you can take practical steps today to enhance your metabolic health and increase your chances of living a longer, healthier life.

12.5 The Future of Preventive Healthcare

Preventive healthcare is rapidly evolving, driven by advances in technology, genetics, and data analytics. As we move toward a future where healthcare becomes more **proactive** rather than reactive, the goal will be to detect and prevent diseases long before symptoms appear. **Metabolic health**, in particular, will benefit greatly from these developments, as many of the most common and life-threatening conditions—such as diabetes, heart disease, and obesity—are deeply connected to metabolic dysfunction. In this final section, we'll explore how **technology**, **personalization**, and **self-monitoring** will shape the future of preventive healthcare and how you can leverage these advancements to maintain optimal metabolic health.

How Technology Will Shape Preventive Medicine

Technology is already playing a pivotal role in the future of **preventive healthcare**, with **wearables**, **apps**, and **AI-driven platforms** allowing individuals to continuously monitor their health metrics in real time. The ability to track things like **blood glucose**, **heart rate variability**, and **sleep patterns** enables people to catch early signs of metabolic dysfunction long before they manifest as chronic disease.

In the future, we can expect more advanced versions of these technologies, providing deeper insights into metabolic function and disease risk. For example, next-generation **wearables** may integrate data from continuous glucose monitors (CGMs), stress sensors, and gut microbiome analyzers to give you a comprehensive view of your metabolic health. These devices could alert you to early signs of insulin resistance, inflammation, or hormonal imbalances, allowing you to make **lifestyle changes** or seek treatment before these issues develop into more serious conditions.

AI-powered platforms will also enhance preventive healthcare by analyzing the massive amounts of data collected from wearables and medical records. These platforms will not only provide personalized health insights but also predict disease risk with greater accuracy than ever before. For example, an AI-driven app could analyze your long-term data to predict your risk of developing type 2 diabetes within the next five years, then offer tailored recommendations for diet, exercise, and medication to reduce that risk.

Technology will also help shift the focus of healthcare from occasional visits to the doctor to continuous **remote monitoring**. By sharing your health data with healthcare providers through **telemedicine platforms**, you can receive ongoing feedback and adjustments to your health plan based on how your body responds to various interventions. This constant feedback loop will allow for more **precise** and **adaptive** approaches to managing your metabolic health.

The Growing Role of Self-Monitoring in Health Management

In the future, individuals will take greater control of their own healthcare, with **self-monitoring** playing a crucial role in maintaining **metabolic balance**. As we've seen throughout this book, tracking key metrics like **blood sugar**, **cholesterol levels**, and **sleep quality** can help you make data-driven decisions about your diet, exercise, and lifestyle.

Self-monitoring tools, such as continuous glucose monitors and fitness trackers, will become even more integrated into daily life. These devices will become more accurate, user-friendly, and affordable, making them accessible to a wider audience. With the ability to monitor your health in real time, you can take immediate action when something goes awry. For instance, if your glucose levels spike after a meal, you can adjust your diet or activity level accordingly to bring them back into balance.

One of the most significant shifts in preventive healthcare will be the ability to **detect metabolic imbalances** at a cellular level before they manifest as symptoms. Future wearables may even be able to monitor **mitochondrial function** or **hormonal fluctuations**, giving you deeper insights into how your body is operating. By addressing these imbalances early, you can prevent the onset of metabolic diseases like type 2 diabetes or cardiovascular disease.

In addition, **microbiome testing** will become more accessible, allowing individuals to monitor their gut health on a regular basis. Since the gut microbiome plays a significant role in metabolism and inflammation, keeping it balanced will be critical for long-term health. Regular testing can help you adjust your diet or take targeted probiotics to maintain a healthy microbiome, preventing conditions like obesity, insulin resistance, and chronic inflammation.

Trends in Proactive Healthcare for Future Generations

As we look ahead, the focus of healthcare will continue to shift from treatment to **prevention**, particularly when it comes to metabolic health. One of the biggest trends in preventive medicine will be **personalized nutrition** and **precision healthcare**, tailored to an individual's genetic makeup, microbiome, and lifestyle.

Genetic testing will become more commonplace, offering insights into how your DNA influences your metabolic health. For instance, genetic testing might reveal that you have a higher predisposition to insulin resistance or that your body metabolizes carbohydrates differently than the average person. With this information, healthcare providers can offer **customized dietary** and **exercise plans** that align with your specific genetic profile, reducing your risk of metabolic dysfunction.

Another trend that will shape the future of preventive healthcare is the growing use of **predictive analytics**. By analyzing your genetic data alongside lifestyle factors such as diet, exercise, and environmental exposures, predictive analytics can give you a clearer picture of your future health risks. With these insights, you'll be able to make **proactive decisions** to protect your health before problems arise. For example, if predictive analytics reveal a high risk of developing cardiovascular disease, you could adopt a heart-healthy diet, increase physical activity, or start medications early to reduce that risk.

Behavioral coaching is also set to play a major role in preventive healthcare. Future healthcare platforms may include AI-driven coaching that provides real-time advice based on your current health metrics. If your stress levels are high, for example, the AI coach might recommend a breathing exercise or a short walk to lower cortisol and improve insulin sensitivity. This type of immediate feedback helps reinforce healthy behaviors and makes preventive healthcare more actionable.

Finally, **public health initiatives** will likely push for greater awareness around metabolic health and preventive care. Governments and healthcare organizations may incentivize preventive health practices, offering subsidies for wearable technology, gym memberships, or nutrition counseling to encourage healthier lifestyles. By promoting a **preventive mindset** early, future generations will be equipped with the tools and knowledge to manage their metabolic health effectively, reducing the burden of chronic diseases on the healthcare system.

The future of **preventive healthcare** is bright, offering more **personalized**, **data-driven**, and **proactive** approaches to metabolic health. With the integration of technology, genetic insights, and real-time health monitoring, we are moving toward a future where metabolic dysfunction can be detected and managed long before it leads to chronic disease. As these tools become more accessible, individuals will take greater ownership of their health, making informed decisions to protect their metabolic function and extend their healthspan. By embracing these trends, you can ensure that your health remains in balance and that you're always one step ahead of potential issues.

Conclusion

As we come to the end of this journey through the fascinating world of **metabolic health,** I want to take a moment to thank you for investing your time and energy in reading this book. Your commitment to understanding and optimizing your health is truly commendable. The information you've absorbed, the practices you've learned, and the insights you've gained are all vital steps toward improving your well-being and living a longer, healthier, and more fulfilling life.

The concept of **metabolic health** might seem complex, but at its core, it is incredibly empowering. You now know that your metabolism is much more than just how quickly your body burns calories—it's the foundation of your **energy**, **vitality**, and **resilience**. From how you process food to how you respond to stress, sleep, and exercise, your metabolism governs your ability to thrive. And the best part is, you have the tools to influence it. Every meal you eat, every hour of sleep you get, every stress-relief technique you practice, and every step you take has the power to shape your metabolism in profound ways.

What I hope you take away from this book is the knowledge that **you are in control**. You've learned about the importance of **personalized nutrition**, how to improve your metabolic flexibility, the role of **hormonal balance**, and how to optimize your lifestyle through **exercise**, **sleep**, and **stress management**. You've also seen how advances in technology—like **wearables**, **AI**, and **genetic testing**—are making it easier to monitor your health and make informed decisions about how to live your best life. Most importantly, you've learned that **prevention** is key. By understanding and monitoring your metabolic health, you can take proactive steps to prevent many of the chronic diseases that have become all too common in today's world.

But knowledge is only the first step. Now, it's time to put it into action.

A Message of Hope

The journey to better health is not always an easy one. There will be days when the challenges seem overwhelming, when stress takes over, when sleep feels elusive, or when making the healthiest choice feels like an impossible task. But every small decision you make in the right direction adds up over time. **Consistency is key**. Each healthy habit you cultivate, no matter how small, has the power to transform your health in the long run.

This book was written with the hope of **empowering you** to take control of your metabolic health and live with more energy, less illness, and greater clarity. The road to optimal health is a journey, not a destination. You don't need to implement every piece of advice all at once. Start with one or two changes that feel manageable, and build from there. Whether it's improving your diet, introducing more movement into your day, or prioritizing your mental well-being, every step you take brings you closer to the best version of yourself.

And remember, **you are not alone** on this journey. Your health is a lifelong project, and it's okay to ask for help when you need it. Whether it's consulting a healthcare professional, joining a support group, or simply reaching out to friends and family, building a community of support around your goals can make all the difference.

Good Energy for the Future

At the core of this book lies the concept of **good energy**—the fuel that powers our bodies, our minds, and our spirits. When we talk about metabolic health, what we're really talking about is giving your body the tools it needs to produce **good energy**—energy that sustains you through the ups and downs of life, energy that fuels your passions, and energy that allows you to be the healthiest, most vibrant version of yourself.

Good energy isn't just about what we put into our bodies; it's about how we live our lives. It's about cultivating positivity, surrounding ourselves with people who uplift us, engaging in activities that bring us joy, and finding meaning in the everyday. The choices you make today—about what to eat, how to move, how to rest, and how to manage stress—will determine the quality of your energy tomorrow and for years to come.

As you continue on your health journey, remember that **good energy** is not just a goal; it's a way of life. It's about finding balance, nurturing your body, and treating yourself with kindness. And it's about being proactive—because the better we take care of ourselves now, the better our chances of living long, healthy lives filled with vitality.

Bonus Resources to Support Your Journey

As a token of our appreciation for your commitment to improving your health, we're excited to offer **three bonus resources** that we believe will help you along your journey to metabolic wellness. These resources are designed to give you practical tools, actionable tips, and ongoing support as you apply the principles you've learned in this book to your everyday life.

While we'll decide on the exact nature of these bonuses shortly, we can assure you that each one will be carefully curated to maximize your results and keep you moving forward on the path to **good energy**. Whether it's a detailed **meal plan**, a **workout routine** designed to boost metabolism, or a **meditation guide** to help you manage stress and improve sleep, our goal is to equip you with everything you need to succeed.

These bonuses are our way of saying **thank you** for choosing to invest in your health. We believe in the power of this information, and we believe in **you**. You've taken an important step by educating yourself on the ins and outs of metabolic health, and we're confident that with these additional resources, you'll have even more tools to thrive.

The Journey Continues

As you finish this book and move forward, take a moment to reflect on how far you've come. Understanding your metabolism and how to optimize it is a powerful asset, and the knowledge you've gained will serve you well throughout your life. But the journey doesn't end here. The beauty of metabolic health is that it evolves with you. As you age, as your life circumstances change, and as new research emerges, your approach to health will adapt.

The key is to stay curious, stay proactive, and stay committed to your well-being. Continue learning, continue refining your habits, and continue seeking out new ways to support your metabolic health. By doing so, you'll ensure that you not only live longer but also live **better**—with energy, clarity, and vitality.

Remember, **good energy** is within your reach. It's in the food you eat, the way you move, the quality of your sleep, and the strength of your resilience. Every choice you make is an opportunity to fuel your body with the energy it needs to thrive.

Thank you again for joining me on this journey. I hope this book has provided you with valuable insights, actionable advice, and the motivation to take charge of your health. Here's to a future filled with **good energy**, vibrant health, and a lifetime of well-being.

Stay energized, stay healthy, and most importantly—**stay empowered**.

We hope the three **bonus resources** that follow will further support your path to metabolic wellness. Each one has been designed to help you stay on track, whether you're looking for guidance on nutrition, exercise, or stress management. We are excited to share these tools with you, and we believe they will provide the extra boost you need to fully embrace the **good energy** lifestyle.

Thank you for reading, and we wish you continued success on your health journey!

BONUS

Scan me!

Made in the USA
Las Vegas, NV
06 December 2024

13477926R00136